SEX, OR THE UNBEARABLE

A series edited by
Lauren Berlant and
Lee Edelman

SEX, OR THE UNBEARABLE

LAUREN BERLANT AND LEE EDELMAN

DUKE UNIVERSITY PRESS

Durham and London

2014

© 2014 Duke University Press
All rights reserved
Printed in the United States of
America on acid-free paper ∞
Designed by Amy Ruth Buchanan
Typeset in Quadraat by Tseng
Information Systems, Inc.

....

Library of Congress
Cataloging-in-Publication Data
Berlant, Lauren Gail, 1957–
Sex, or the unbearable / Lauren Berlant
and Lee Edelman.
pages   cm — (Theory Q)
Includes bibliographical references and index.
ISBN 978-0-8223-5580-9 (cloth : alk. paper)
ISBN 978-0-8223-5594-6 (pbk. : alk. paper)
1. Sex. 2. Queer theory. 3. Intimacy (Psychology)
I. Edelman, Lee, 1953– II. Title. III. Series:
Theory Q.
HQ75.15.B47 2014
306.7—dc23   2013025531

CONTENTS

....

PREFACE

....

Sex, or the Unbearable: the title of this book does not offer its readers a choice between these two terms, as in "your money, or your life." Nor does it mean to imply that we think of sex as reducible to "the unbearable." To be honest, there's not that much sex in the book either, and the "unbearable" to which it points is all crossed over with the enjoyable too. But then again, enjoyment itself, as we discuss it here, can be unbearable. What we offer instead is an analysis of relations that both overwhelm and anchor us — an affective paradox that often shapes the experience of sex. We approach sex here as a site, therefore, at which relationality is invested with hopes, expectations, and anxieties that are often *experienced* as unbearable. Sex, though subject to the pressures of legal sanction, social judgment, unconscious drives, and contradictory desires, holds out the prospect of discovering new ways of being and of being in the world. But it also raises the possibility of confronting our limit in ourselves or in another, of being inundated psychically or emotionally. *Sex, or the Unbearable* examines our attempts to remain rooted in the social by both holding fast to and moving beyond our accustomed ways of experiencing ourselves and our connectedness to others. It explores the forms of negotiation we resort to in dealing with intimate estrangement, and it tries to enact, in its own formal structure, the constant, and at times disconcerting, adjustments those forms of negotiation demand.

The following chapters approach the scene of relationality by focusing on the "negativity" that can make it so disturbing. Negativity for us refers to the psychic and social incoherences and divisions, conscious and unconscious alike, that trouble any totality or fixity of identity. It denotes, that is, the relentless force that unsettles the fantasy of sovereignty. But its effects, in our view, are not just negative, since negativity unleashes the energy that allows for the possibility of change. So too "nonsovereignty," a term to which we'll return, invokes the psychoanalytic notion of the subject's constitutive division that keeps us, as subjects, from fully knowing or being in control of ourselves and that prompts our misrecognition of our own motives and desires. At the same time, nonsovereignty invokes a political idiom and tradition, broadly indicating questions of self-control, autonomy, and the constraints upon them. To encounter ourselves as nonsovereign, we suggest, is to encounter relationality itself, in the psychic, social, and political senses of the term. For that reason, this book attends to those moments when negativity disturbs the presumption of sovereignty by way of "an encounter," specifically, an encounter with the estrangement and intimacy of being in relation. Sex is exemplary in the way it powerfully induces such encounters, but such encounters exceed those experiences we recognize as sex.

These dialogues explore such encounters while simultaneously recording and performing one. It could be no other way. Relationality always includes a scenic component, a fantasmatic staging. It puts into play reaction, accommodation, transference, exchange, and the articulation of narratives. Just what an encounter entails, however, remains for us unresolved. As it must. For an encounter refers to an episode, an event, its fantasmatic scene, and the myriad misrecognitions that inform the encounter and define its limit. Our various ways of theorizing such encounters with relation shape our different views of the political and affective consequences of social embeddedness. We are constantly asking, What do our distinctive responses to each other and our cases tell us about the structural conditions that produce the encounter with nonsovereignty in the first place?

Though the negativity inseparable from the sexual encounter comes to the fore most insistently in the final chapter of this book, it makes itself felt repeatedly in the dialogues that follow. For encounter in all its ambiguity shapes the experience of sex, giving rise to various forms of response, including, as the first two chapters suggest, optimism and reparativity. We wonder throughout these dialogues whether it is possible to endure the experience of relation in the absence of optimism for bearing or surmounting what overwhelms us in ourselves and in each other. Is optimism, in fact, invariably at work in negativity? Or, conversely, is optimism a disavowal of what's unbearable in negativity? Do we even mean the same thing by optimism? This book attempts to hold such questions steadily in view. Even where we disagree with each other in the ways that we address them, though, we proceed together through the breaks and divisions that enable conversation, politics, and the creation of new social forms.

Sex, or the Unbearable is thus an experiment in the forms of theoretical production. It proceeds from the belief that dialogue may permit a powerful approach to negativity, since dialogue has some of the risk and excitement we confront in the intimate encounter. Not for nothing does the OED list "communication" and "conversation" as the primary meanings of *intercourse*. In its dialogic structure, then, this book takes shape as collaboration, argument, and exploration at once. It belongs to an experimental genre in which theory, politics, and close textual analysis encounter the pedagogical necessity of responding to the provocations of otherness. Dialogue commits us to grappling with negativity, nonsovereignty, and social relation not only as abstract concepts but also as the substance and condition of our responses—and our responsibilities—to each other.

Reimagining forms of relation entails imagining new genres of experience. These chapters try to extend the generic contours of theoretical writing by making exchange, dialogic give-and-take, a genuine form of encounter. By that we mean that throughout this book we try to attend not only to what we can readily agree upon but also to what remains opaque or unpersuasive about the other's ideas, what threatens to block or stymie us. Resistance, misconstruction, frustration, anxiety, becoming defensive, feeling misunderstood: we see these as central to our engagement with each other and to our ways of confronting the challenge of negativity and encounter. Far from construing such responses as failures in the coherence or economy of our dialogues, we consider them indispensable to our efforts to think relationality. An academic culture in the United States still dominated by the privilege of the monograph only rarely affords occasions for critics to converse with each other in print. That may reflect conversation's low place in the hierarchy of literary genres. Structurally determined by interruption, shifts in perspective, metonymic displacements, and the giving up of control, conversation complicates the prestige of autonomy and the fiction of authorial sovereignty by introducing the unpredictability of moving in relation to another. One never can know in advance to what one's interlocutor will respond or what turns the conversation may take through the associations of a single word. We are aware that what we're saying here sounds a lot like what we say about sex—and that, of course, is the point. As the book proceeds, the structural resonances among sex, politics, and theory become ever more insistently the focus of our analysis.

This discussion starts, as all discussions do, in the middle of many idioms and vernaculars and at the point where many genealogies converge. Entering a conversation always means entering it with an idiolect that has to adjust to someone else's, difficult as that may be. As a consequence, our own conversation includes and exceeds us at once; references taken for granted by one person are foreign to another; historical contexts or philosophical grounds are never fully shared (nor could they be, given the infinite expansion of knowledge that would require); alignments of context or reference take shape simultaneously as gaps, missed encounters, and blockages. So the process of clarification on which we embark must operate immanently from within the conversation rather than by appealing to an objectivized understanding of a set of issues that the conversation unproblematically presupposes. Each of us offers a set of terms that start to look different when the other uses them, and each of us develops ways of testing out, querying, and accounting for the other's conceptualizations. This process might make any reader, including the writers themselves, desire some dictionary or reference point to stabilize the conversation or long for an accompanying seminar to fill in the gaps and provide us with background knowledge to make the going smoother. But conversation, like relationality, proceeds in the absence of such a reference point or undisputed ground, often, in fact, producing the fiction of that ground only retroactively.

The question of assumed knowledge can also manifest itself as a question of address. Any given reader may feel that the conversation is taking place elsewhere, failing to address her or him, or that it shifts its address unpredictably from inclusion to exclusion. Being in relation invariably involves the animation of distance and closeness; in that sense even direct address can be felt as indirect and acknowledgment can seem like misrecognition. Both of us had that experience in the course of these conversations, and it would be surprising if our readers did not have it too. But the process of negotiating those shifts, of finding one's bearings, is at the center of the ongoing project of relationality we explore in this text.

To sustain the critical dialogue we put fidelity to our ideas and their consequences above the performance of our friendship, on the one hand, or the scoring of points, on the other. (Whether or not we succeed, of course, is not for us to say.) Though friendship serves as the ground from which these dialogues arise, it doesn't prompt us to deny our differences or obscure our intellectual or political commitments. At the same time, those commitments themselves are what these dialogues put to the test. In the course of these conversations we both experienced clarification, surprise, and, most important, transformation; there were moments, that is, when the contours of our own understandings noticeably shifted and something of the other's language or intellectual imperatives affected our own. The differences in our political and theoretical investments did not, of course, disappear, but something else, new ways of inhabiting those investments, appeared as well.

For all the insistence of such differences, though, we acknowledge at the outset that we came to these dialogues with similar intellectual backgrounds and theoretical allegiances. Some might see that as a limitation, a failure of the dialogue to allow for an encounter with the disturbances of multiple kinds of difference. But even in the narrowcast of an encounter with the similar we recognize no putative sameness of self, no sovereignty, no coherence, and no identity that doesn't reveal its *own* radical differences. To be sure, many other encounters than this one both could and should take place—and encounters with other sorts of difference than those that develop here. But one of the points this book hopes to make is that any encounter (with the world, with another, or even with oneself) discloses a nest of differences that carry what Barbara Johnson so memorably called "the surprise of otherness" (1987, 16).

One of our goals, as we've already mentioned, is to think together about the social, political, and theoretical consequences of "negativity." Negativity points to many kinds of relation in what follows, from the unbearable, often unknowable, psychic conflicts that constitute the subject to the social forms of negation that also, but differently, produce subjectivity. Generally negativity signifies a resistance to or undoing of the stabilizing frameworks of coherence imposed on thought and lived experience. In its disturbance of such totalizations, negativity enacts the dissent without which politics disappears. Negativity, in this sense, is inseparable from the struggles of subordinated persons to resist the social conditions of their devaluation. However, by challenging the coherence of the categories through which the subordinated produce their claims for legitimation, negativity can also become an obstacle to their organized resistance to things as they are. This double valence of negativity accounts for its centrality to a set of debates that have occupied queer theory for some time—and that occupy our debate with each other here.

One of the motives for our orientation toward questions of negativity and relation is to dislodge one position in those debates, what has been called "the antisocial thesis," from a set of understandable anxieties that it has provoked among some queer thinkers.[1] The historic practice of LGBTQ studies has been toward reclaiming and repairing lost histories and ongoing practices of delegitimation. Negativity as a source for social theory tends to reject the impulses to repair social relations that appear to us irreparable, and in that light, our work might seem quietistic, apolitical, nihilist, defeatist, or even irresponsible. By engaging closely with sociality and with our own deep-rooted tendencies to think about its zones of optimism and longing, we are seeking to make a persuasive case for the necessity of recognizing the importance of addressing structural antagonisms in any analytic of the social. In doing so, we seek to affirm negativity's central role in any antinormative politics. We hope this conversation might permit a reframing of the antisocial

1. While evidence of that debate abounds, the most concentrated venue of its performance can be found in the PMLA roundtable "The Antisocial Thesis in Queer Theory."

thesis that has already generated such lively debate and so much important theoretical work by its critics and adherents alike.

Part of the problem we have to confront in trying to move that debate forward, however, is that the very name "antisocial" disregards our persistent embeddedness in and attentiveness to sociality. It is not a matter for either of us of standing outside the social or sociality or against the possibility of creating more capacious social worlds. Rather we recognize that negativity emerges as resistance to the fixity of social forms that seem to define the possibilities for and the limits of relationality. We want to explore the valences of social intensities and fantasies, of the contradictory pressures implicit in established forms of relation, in order to read them not in any simple antithesis to the social but rather as intrinsic to it.

We recognize too that "antisocial" has sometimes functioned as a synonym or coded shorthand for "antisentimental" or "antireparative." Where the issues of sentimentality and repair are concerned, our positions are not identical and we do not agree in all cases on the meanings of those terms. These dialogues address them directly, though, and try to work through the ways we understand the investments they bespeak. Nor do we exempt ourselves from investments, including unrecognized investments, in what those terms may name. Our approach, however, depends on acknowledging the specific contexts of their uses in order to recognize both what they enable and what they might foreclose. This book thus aspires to reformulate discussion of the antisocial thesis by conceding from the outset that the questions of sociality so vigorously argued in its wake are genuinely hard and politically imperative, which is why they call forth such intensity of thought on all sides of the debate.

It is in the context of that debate that we came to put this book together. Having mounted different but related arguments against the normative domination of sex, sexuality, and political collectivity by the ideological lure of the future, we were separately called on by Heather Love to give papers at a conference, Rethinking Sex (2009), that she was organizing in honor of Gayle Rubin. Initially invited to give papers at a session tentatively called "Tomorrow," we decided instead to have a public conversation that would build on Rubin's writings in order to move beyond the accounts of futurity we each had separately produced and engage instead the implication of sex in the normative logic of optimism. We began with the notion of optimism because it hooks us to fantasies of the good life, however the good life may be defined. Often such optimism enacts the hope of successful integration into dominant orders—social, psychic, and political—by anticipating ways of resolving the various contradictions amid which we live. Sex, as a locus for optimism, is a site at which the promise of overcoming division and antagonism is frequently played out. But the consequences of such efforts to resolve our social and psychic contradictions can include the establishment of sexual norms and the circumscription of sex for socially legitimated ends. It can equally, however, give rise to fantasies of sexual liberation and a paradise of polymorphous sexualities. We have different concerns about the effects and efficacy of these fantasies, which led us to wonder what it would mean to think about or even desire the experience of sex without optimism. What if we accepted the challenge of negativity and began the process of conceptualizing sex in the absence of such optimism? What sorts of displacements would it introduce into our ways of thinking sex?

That first conversation challenged clichés about the antisocial thesis by making criticism a social and collaborative form even while broaching sociality and sex outside their connection to repair. Our presentation at the Rethinking Sex conference, the basis for chapter 1, undertook to show that negativity, far from being reductively antisocial, is invariably an aspect of the social: that sociality's inherent contradictions give rise to structures of self-relation fundamentally out of synch with themselves. We began with a common interest in negativity's resistance to forms of sovereignty and so in its status as an impediment to normativity's will to social closure and coherence. Our discussion touched on the tragic, dramatic, and comic frames that negativity can inhabit and surprisingly (to us) found its focal objects in the vistas of "the queer adorable." The energy informing that dialogue emerged from our efforts to be in relation at once to each other, our objects, and our ideas, while unfolding the negativity of relation as indispensable to political vitality.

In the aftermath of that conversation, finding ourselves still working through the questions that it raised, we began to ask if it would be useful to try to expand it into a book. So when we were invited the following year to take part in a panel at the annual convention of the Modern Language Association that was being organized in memory of our friend and colleague, Eve Kosofsky Sedgwick, we decided once more to use the opportunity to pursue these ideas together. Sedgwick's work, over the arc of her career, inspired us to return to the ideological imbrications of sex and the forms of optimism, but to do so by engaging negativity in the context of her analyses of repair.

Given the inevitable, and often unbearable, disturbances onto which sex can open, how is it possible, we asked ourselves (and each other and Sedgwick as well), to address that negativity as inseparable from what is most compelling in sex? In pursuing this thought we had to deal with the difficulty of articulating the join of psychic and social scenes and dynamics. Any analytic encounter with sex should push psychoanalytic accounts of the subject and of the subject's psychic experience to acknowledge and address their constitution within an invariably political field. Sedgwick's interest in Silvan Tomkins and Melanie Klein—especially as her theoretical and activist concerns intersected with her own therapeutic ambitions in *A Dialogue on Love*—encouraged us to tackle a question that followed directly from our previous dialogue: Can we hope to transform our relation to the structural disturbance of the subject's coherence without just producing ever new fantasies of simplifying or repairing it? Our efforts to respond to the challenge posed by such ruptures of continuity gave shape to the talk that later became our second chapter, "What Survives." Sedgwick's death, which viscerally brought home the insistence of rupture in relation, impelled us to explore what follows—affectively, narratively, and politically—from the persistence of negativity in every practice of repair.

Among the responses that greeted our presentation of "What Survives" were several that wondered how to survive the irreparable negativity it evoked. The possibility of a life not governed by the logic of repair seemed, according to some in the audience, unbearable to imagine. How, in the absence of wanting to repair, could one possibly go on? What would such going on look like if we turned our theory into practice? Would living with negativity entail the death of the optimism that animates desire and energizes politics? We felt a responsibility to address these questions as clearly as possible and to flesh out the imbrication of negativity, politics, and the phenomenality of life in order to show how negativity is not the opposite of politics, not a practice of withdrawal from contesting the terms or structures of existence, but rather a challenge to engage with politics in unexpected places and in unpredicted ways.

We also felt the need to think about theory as a type of social practice and to consider the aesthetic in terms of the narratives with which we turn life to account. In the first chapter we focused on separate aesthetic (and, in each case, visually iconic) objects through which to organize our speculations on what sex without optimism might mean. In the second we used Sedgwick's texts to approach what's beyond the optimistic model of attachment forms meant to solve the problem of living. What survives once the model of reparative relation is forced to share space with all sorts of negativity or when it starts to open onto a negativity of its own? For the final chapter we thought it important to link the question of *living* with negativity to the processes of *narrating* it, gathering up the diverse kinds of realism, causality, fantasy, and organization in movement that narrative forces to the fore. It struck us as crucial, in that regard, to engage a common text, one that would somehow speak to the question of living with negativity while opening onto the interrelations among sex, narrative, and the prospect for changing how we inhabit and relate to the world.

After considering a wide array of objects that might galvanize our thought, we read Lydia Davis's Collected Stories together and knew we had found our author. Though drawn to a dozen of Davis's texts, each perfect for this chapter's project, we decided to direct our energies to a close reading of only one. A single text seemed fitting here because this chapter, following our speculations on repair in "What Survives," concerns finding ways of living with an object, or with the loss or breakdown of an object, that roots one in the world.

"Break It Down," the story we finally chose, engages living with others and living on in their absence. Enigmatic and haunting, filled with the pathos of a narrator not fully controlling what he reveals, "Break It Down" provides a scaffold for this chapter's meditations on negativity. It does so, moreover, while enacting a continuous interrogation of what "sex" means. Because it plays so crucial a role in "Living with Negativity" and because we want it to enter our conversation here in its own right, we have reprinted "Break It Down" as an appendix to our dialogue with the generous approval of Lydia Davis and the permission of her publishers. In this way we hope the story makes audible another voice in this book and provides the opportunity for another encounter with Davis's work—an encounter different, we hope, from reading the story in a different context and one that adds a different context to the dialogues gathered here.

....

We have suggested that this book uses dialogue to refine theoretical questions and to bring different aesthetic and critical archives to bear upon them. Those questions about the overwhelming intensities that shape ordinary subjectivity, even in noncrisis times, are harder than any one dialogue can bear, and we are not seeking *to do justice* to them, in the sense of repairing the world in which they operate as registers of subjectivity and power—if, that is, repair and justice could ever be construed as synonymous. We aim instead, through our own conversation, to initiate many others, including one among theorists of politics, affect, psychoanalysis, and aesthetics, that would try to account for the disturbances and anchors within relationality (to ourselves, across ourselves, to the world at large) and for the effects those disturbances and anchors have on our thinking about sociality. We believe that such conversations can expand our sense of sociality and the possibility of political movement. Paradoxically, though, our strategy of enlargement relies on narrowing our focus here. In other work we each might have moved outward to different exempla and archives. Here the form of the dialogue impels us to ever greater specificity as we respond to a recurrent anxiety about whether our iterations of words, objects, and scenes are understood in the way we intended. Along with the disturbance it occasions, though, the dialogue form affords us the chance to experience the "same thing" as different and to encounter the metamorphic potential that the sameness of things contains. Ultimately for us, it isn't a choice between disturbance and transformational possibility. We are interested in the inseparability of the two, in what can never be predicted or controlled in any engagement with the world, with otherness, and thus with ourselves as well.

1. SEX WITHOUT OPTIMISM

LAUREN BERLANT: Because many of us—I'm not presuming universality here—want so much from sex, from the study of sex, and from activism that foregrounds countering erotophobia, and because so many of us want relief from rage and pessimism about sex too, a phrase like "sex without optimism" might raise hackles. It might sound like a program that advocates coolness, being above the fray, a dare to not care, an affective or emotional imperative, or disrespect for optimism. I can assure you that we are not advocating for any of this.

LEE EDELMAN: Like the book for which it stands as the gateway, this chapter finds its origin more in questions than in answers—questions that Lauren and I have been trying to think about together. In large part those questions center on the very concept of togetherness. They impel us to interrogate the practices, effects, and ideologies of relation both in terms of the others with whom we find ourselves variously together (socially, erotically, politically, spatially, categorically, economically, ecologically) and in terms of the self that may (or may not) claim a unity or togetherness of its own. We approach the issue of relationality through the rubric of "sex without optimism" because sex, for us, whatever else it may signify or be made to figure, denotes an encounter with otherness that attains the stability of knowable relation only by way of an optimism that erases its negativity.

Jacques Lacan's well-known assertion that "there is no sexual relation" resists the imperative to resolve the structural antagonism of the Symbolic (given a contingent expression in heteronormativity's sexual binarism) through the fantasy, and so the optimism, of a successfully realized relation (Lacan 1991/2007, 116). Lacan, that is, attends to what is negative and unknowable in sex insofar as sexual difference eludes every effort to comprehend it. Such a reference to Lacan, more pertinent perhaps to my approach than to Lauren's, might help nonetheless to crystallize what seems inseparable from sex for both of us: the encounter with what exceeds and undoes the subject's fantasmatic sovereignty. Against the specific optimism such a fantasy bespeaks, sex affords a privileged site for encountering negativity—a negativity that registers at once the insistence of enjoyment, of the drive, and of various disturbances that inhere in relation itself.

LB: Negativity, the "without" in our title, magnetizes many different things, and one of our aims throughout this volume is to elaborate on the richness and incoherence of the concept (if you add up all of the things each of us means). But briefly, by negativity I am pointing at once to the self-cleaving work of the drives, being socially oppressed, and being nonsovereign, affectively undone by being in relation. It's worth saying, therefore, that nonsovereignty and negativity are not precise synonyms (like most synonyms or proposals of likeness, they also imply a world of differences): the latter derives from a philosophical and psychoanalytic engagement, while the former derives from traditions in political theory that traverse social and affective relationality. The main political question is how we understand and mobilize the relations among these concepts, phenomena, and structures.

But it's hard to stay focused on the *variety* when the affective impact of attention to the subject's negativity so often reads as nihilistic or just anti-x when we mean something more overdetermined and dynamic. For example, I don't think that "sex . . . attains the stability of knowable relation only by way of an optimism that erases its negativity": what it means to know, what it means to want what's not knowable in advance or controllable, what it means to sense something without knowing it, does not add up to amnesia, foreclosure, disavowal, or erasure—but neither does erasure itself, as Lee's writing in this chapter will soon attest. Can understanding more about the many ways that sexuality manifests itself as nonsovereignty, radical incoherence, and a scene both for optimism and subordination transform what sexuality stands for and does?

So we came up with the phrase "sex without optimism" and then had to figure out what we meant.

LE: One way to tell our story is by starting with the problem of story as such and considering how telling it is that we tell our stories here so differently. However attenuated, qualified, ironized, interrupted, or deconstructed it may be, a story implies a direction; it signals, as story, a movement that leads toward some payoff or profit, some comprehension or closure, however open-ended. This leading *toward* necessarily entails a correlative "leading *from*," the "leading from" or "out of" at the root of "education." Even in those moments when we imagine ourselves immersed in its permanent middle, the story, so conceived at least, moves through time toward its putative end, where it seems to define the field within which it produces its sense of sense. Absent that framework of expectation, it isn't a story at all, just metonymic associations attached to a given nucleus.

But even such an elaboration would return us to the conventions of story: the refusal of story will always enact the story of its refusal. This orientation toward a future, toward something always yet to come, conceived as bestowing a value on life by way of the future anterior, by way of the life one *will have lived*, conceived, moreover, as justifying this refusal to live it *while one could*: this is what I call optimism, a condition so wide in its reach that it shapes our experience into narratives touched with the gloss we might think of as finish, in more than one sense of that term. To the extent that such optimism aspires to the finish of this universal gloss, we might view it as truly Panglossian and acknowledge the extent to which it compels a regulatory discipline that, with apologies to Michel Foucault, we could designate as Panoptimism.

Our conversation begins as an attempt to think about how to be pro-sex without succumbing to Panoptimism, or even to the sort of sexual optimism implicit in sexual liberation—and to do so by thinking about alternatives to narrative knowledge and knowledge as narrative: to do so, that is, by once again, as Gayle Rubin recommended, rethinking sex and posing it over and against education as a "leading out" of ignorance, inability, and bewilderment and into the condition of mastery, understanding, and realized sovereignty. As sex, in this context, compels the provisionality of relation, so the dialogue toward which we are moving neither affirms our shared identity nor reifies our differences. It puts those differences into play instead, bringing them into focus at one moment and revising the optic the next so that openings onto areas of agreement also make visible new zones of dissent. That play bespeaks the enjoyment we take, the goad or provocation we find, in one another's work, and it aims to allow for the sorts of surprises, interruptions, and recalibrations that come, or don't, with thinking in the absence of predetermined outcomes.

Nothing was certain as we began this project; nothing was fixed in advance. We still don't even know for sure that we mean the same things by "sex." For me, it has something to do with experiencing corporeally, and in the orbit of the libidinal, the shock of discontinuity and the encounter with nonknowledge. But versions of such an encounter will inform the movement of these dialogues too, which may induce, libidinally or not, some shocks of discontinuity as well. Together, in the cross-cut meditations, observations, and questions that determine their shape, these dialogues will reverse education's leading out and return to the place of sex in thought, or rather, in thought's multiplication: in its doubling, that is, by the two of us and by the doubling back implicit in the process of re-thinking. As one might expect from a critical mode that dabbles in doubling back, we abandon all hope at the outset of moving toward any definable end. But we're also mindful that such a claim may itself be a form of Panoptimism.

LB: We came to the question of sex without optimism focusing on the ways that sex undoes the subject, but we use idioms that aren't identical, as I suggested: Lee emphasizing the structuring force of jouissance and me emphasizing the activity of affect phenomeno-logically and in historical context—and that matters, as we will see. But we both engage critically the ways that heteronormativity attempts to snuff out libidinal unruliness by projecting evidence of it onto what Rubin calls "sexual outlaws" and other populations deemed excessively appetitive, casting them as exemplary moral and political threats that must be framed, shamed, monitored, and vanquished if the conventional good life, with its "productive" appetites, is going to endure (Rubin 2011, 131). The question we debate remains what else to do with the knowledge of the overwhelming force of sex and drive.

Thus we have both rejected projects of queer optimism that try to repair the subject's negativity into a grounding experiential positivity. Where Lee is concerned, this set of aversions and commitments has been called "the antisocial turn" in queer theory and has turned into a controversy about what embracing negativity must mean, can mean, should mean for people's imaginaries of power and about how to live. Indeed the critique of optimism as foreclosure he recounts has seemed (mistakenly) to some like a critique of imagining life as worth attaching to at all.

But in my advocacy for thinking about the subject as that which is structurally nonsovereign in a way that's intensified by sex, intimacy building, and structural inequality, I have not been accused of being antisocial, just socially awkward, a whole different problem, resulting in a theoretical idiom more slapstick than stentorian, more concerned with the force and impact of what Lee calls "just metonymic associations." This means that, while he focuses on "story" as *always* enacting negativity's drama of expectation and refusal, I am more concerned with that muddled middle where survival and threats to it engender social forms that transform the habitation of negativity's multiplicity, without necessarily achieving "story" in his terms (Berlant 2007). For, you know, I am a utopian, and Lee is not. I do not see optimism primarily as a glossing over, as "fantasy" in the negative sense of resistance to the Real. I am interested in optimism as a mode of attachment to life. I am committed to the political project of imagining how to detach from lives that don't work and from worlds that negate the subjects that produce them; and I aim, along with many antinormative activists, to expand the field of affective potentialities, latent and explicit fantasies, and infrastructures for how to live beyond survival, toward flourishing not later but in the ongoing now. Lee has said to me, as we've built this conversation, that he finds this orientation too close to the kind of be-goodenness that we are also contesting (Berlant 2011).

I would also not describe the negativity of sex and sexuality as Lee just did, as "the shock of discontinuity and the encounter with nonknowledge." That is because I think that subjects are not usually shocked to discover their incoherence or the incoherence of the world; they often find it comic, feel a little ashamed of it, or are interested in it, excited by it, and exhausted by it too, by the constant pressure to adjust that is at the heart of being nonsovereign, subjected to the inconstancy and contingency that they discover in and around themselves. At the same time, people protect their sexual incoherence, and it's worth noticing how they defend the ways that they are unreliable to their self-idealization and their internal noise, including their tangled conceptions of who should have sexual freedom and what kind. Shock, comparatively, is rare.

Finally, in my view, the affective experience of sexual or any nonknowledge is not usually a blockage or limit but is actually the experience of the multiplication of knowledges that have an awkward relation to each other, crowd each other out, and create intensities that require management. This is one place where the desire to cement sex to optimism arises, as any conventionality in the penumbra of sex provides relief from the ordinary muddles that arise in the intimate zones of encounter with other persons and the world. But even the enjoyment of an optimistic reprieve from being overwhelmed within sexualization is not the same thing as the desire for it to be repaired, to go away as a problem, or to achieve a flat consistency. Relief, play, interruption, glitchiness: these can provide a space of interest within which other rhythms and therefore forms of encounter with and within sexuality can be forged.

In short, our commonalities are in our fundamental belief that normativity is an attempt to drown out the subject's constitution by and attachment to varieties of being undone and our strong interest in a pedagogy that does not purchase space for negativity by advocating for a simplifying optimism. I tend to expand from the multiplicities and disjunctures of the affective register within which subjectification is experienced (whether or not recognized as an experience), while Lee focuses even more abstractly on the frameworks of meaning making that require such domination. I tend to dedramatize the experience of being a sexual subject in the ordinary, while Lee sees the subject's reeling experience of his subjective negativity as a drama that becomes dramatized. So we thought that perhaps we should look at different registers of aesthetic mediation that might get both at what we don't share and what we do — a view of the subject's undoing and the wrongheadedness of any reparative politics that turns being undone into a symptom of an illness or a measure of injustice.

....

Initially we thought the phrase "sex without optimism" was very funny. At the same time it pointed toward a difficult project of displacing sex and sexuality from their seesaw status as either causes of or repairs for the precarity of life. But did we really want sex without optimism? Why didn't we just want sex without stupid or destructive optimism? Our divergence in even understanding these questions was most starkly manifested aesthetically. I wanted each of us to curate a montage of sex without optimism. We made a list of films that we thought would provide some examples.

LE: And then things started to get complicated. The more examples we proposed of what we could think of as sex without optimism, whether or not we qualified that optimism as stupid or destructive or cruel, the more it became clear that we didn't necessarily mean the same things by "sex" and that we were finding it hard to locate representations of sex that weren't optimistic. Something, perhaps the aesthetic framing of our various representations, or perhaps the persistence of narrative in the project of reading as such, recurrently seemed to neutralize resistance to Panoptimism's imperative.

Given her investment in thinking about options for sustaining lives that confront the obstacles of an unpropitious present, Lauren's examples tended toward instances in which surviving the dominations of power shaped a narrative about enduring or negotiating the experience of delegitimated being. Given my own suspicion of rhetorics that privilege viability or survival, a suspicion that marks less a difference from Lauren than a difference in inflection, I tended toward instances that depicted a *structure* I associated with sex without optimism (Edelman 2011). For both of us, whatever our definitions of "sex," this meant turning to the distinctive undoing within it — an undoing that we don't see identically but one that we recognize as undoing our own as well as the other's understanding of it. That undoing is not, I must hasten to add, simply or "ultimately" productive. It doesn't move us toward final synthesis or overcome our differences. And it doesn't give us comfort, as if it were an absolute good in itself. It prompts us instead to interrogate the relation of sex to our notions of the good and to consider the "re" in rethinking as repetition and undoing at once and so as bound to the problematic of the drive as we encounter it in sex. I take Lauren's point to heart, after all, when she says that subjects are not generally shocked by the experience of their own incoherence and that what matters most may not, in fact, be blockages or encounters with nonknowledge but the multiplication and overlap of *incompatible* knowledges. But the persistence of that incompatibility, the constant obtrusion of what our will to relational management ignores, denies, or misrecognizes, makes undoing as such the condition of living in a world that is not our own.

If relation exists as a pathway between entities in a multidimensional network wherein those entities themselves are the products of particular sets of relations, then moving across those dimensions and through its infinite relational web will entail an undoing we may not want to experience or acknowledge as such. Shock, as Benjamin taught us, can itself be part of the everyday as well as an exceptional experience of radically traumatizing discontinuity. Even in its everyday form, though, the shock we encounter retains the *potential* to undo our faith in our own ongoingness, our sense of our consistency as subjects (however inconsistently conceived), and to obtrude with an incoherence we cannot master by finding it comic or resolve through the judgment of shame. The corollary to that encounter is anxiety, whose intensities we never fully manage since they signal our too-near approach to what we're driven to enjoy. That's why sex gets invested with such a weighty burden of optimism *as well as* with an often overwhelming burden of anxiety: the closer we come to enjoyment, the greater our need to defend against it—to defend our putative sovereignty against the negativity that empties it out.

Though I agree, then, that incoherence may often feel all too familiar and, in consequence, not shocking at all, my claim is that this very familiarity may testify to the will to domesticate the encounter with what can *never* be made familiar, what escapes our recognized feelings, eluding recognition precisely by virtue of those *recognized* feelings themselves. What I find so compelling about Lauren's attentiveness to the taxonomies of unaccommodated being is the care with which she traces the conditions impelling subjects to normalizing narratives of emotional adequation even while she attends so shrewdly to the strategies by which alternative possibilities for world-building might also begin to emerge. My own imperative remains, however, to question the ground of those possibilities, to question our desire for those possibilities, to the extent that they still remain rooted in the willful management of affective intensities and susceptible, therefore, to the misrecognitions that reify the subject's self, even if the self that the subject reifies is construed as incoherent. The familiarity of incoherence can become a way of denying it. The I that "knows" its incoherence, or has grown accustomed to it, has usually succeeded, if painfully, in the labor of normalizing a self, even when it conceives that self as inadequate to the norm. So for me, the structuring incoherences that queer the self as the center of consciousness, and so of a pseudo-sovereignty, remain unavailable to the subject except in rare moments of traumatic encounter, moments when the potential for shock gets activated by the nearness of the unbearable, which is to say, of our own enjoyment: the enjoyment "we" never own.

Lauren would see the word "traumatic" as an instance of my making grandiose what she invites us to dedramatize, while I would worry that dedramatization is the emptying out, the attempt to neutralize the force of that encounter itself. Not always—and not in Lauren's work—but maybe in our normative relations to ourselves as continuous or viable subjects. Our world-building can't protect us against the worlds that others build, which may or may not have room for us or find us consistent with their survival. Nor can we be sure that the worlds *we* build don't work against our own flourishing. That doesn't mean we could simply choose to forgo the world-building project, any more than we could simply choose to forgo the optimism of attachment, only that it finds its supplement in thinking the encounter with what resists it, producing thereby the problem of relation these dialogues will confront. The negativity of encounter inhabits relation for Lauren and me alike.

But it does so across differences in intellectual tradition and critical vocabulary that Lauren and I must negotiate as we try to move in relation to each other while wrestling with relation as a concept. Lauren's focus on affect leads her to resist my account of sex as the confrontation with a limit; she sees it as "the multiplication of knowledges that have an awkward relation to each other, crowd each other out, and create overwhelmed intensities that require management." What I find of interest, however, beyond the necessity of affect management produced by the multiplication of knowledges are the moments that signal the failure or even the inadequacy of knowledge as such, moments when the frameworks of knowing are not simply incoherently at odds with each other but incapable of accommodating the encounter with something unnamable in the terms they offer and irreducible to relation.

This nonrelation that's internal to relation and that threatens to overwhelm our attempts to manage it by *reasserting* relation is central to my approach to the encounter and to my reading of its structure. The insuperable otherness of this nonrelation finds expression in the negativity that marks the subject's encounter with nonsovereignty, but it escapes the sort of recognition by which the subject could assume that nonsovereignty as something of its own rather than as something that disappropriates it of ownership of itself. Nonsovereignty, as we both agree, is not one thing but many; the nonsovereignty the subject can recognize (and so try to manage, at least affectively) differs from the nonsovereignty manifest, for example, by the drive, by the unconscious, or by the Real that dissolves the consistency of reality as known.

In this regard I would want to define one difference between Lauren's perspective and mine by focusing on her distinction between my engagement with "negativity's drama of expectation and refusal" and her concern with "that muddled middle where survival and threats to it engender social forms that transform the habitation of negativity's multiplicity." Lauren's work directs our attention to the scenic potential of what can seem an immutable relation to oneself, one's objects, or one's world. Her subtle readings of "social forms" and their susceptibility to change, however, differ from my own investment in reading the repetitions of the nonrelation that structures and necessitates those changes. Inherent in the proliferation of social forms lies what structures the social *as* form: the void of the nonrelation that in-forms, which is to say, forms from within, the imperative to formalize relation even while deforming it as well. I tend to focus on the consequences of this antagonism inherent in social forms, while Lauren tends to theorize the social as the site for more scenic sorts of relation, exploring the various ways of inhabiting an environment or of being in the world. But I don't construe this difference in optic or emphasis as absolute. We both attend to the pressure of structures, and we both are committed to thinking about change, even if those notions of structure and change must open to include, in the course of our discussion, the different ways we construe them.

Lauren calls herself a utopian, which she links to the double project of "imagining how to detach from lives that don't work" and expanding what she calls the "field of fantasies" for "flourishing . . . in the ongoing now." I am not a utopian, though I too cast my vote for flourishing. But then I don't see "flourishing" as radically distinct from the experience of "lives that don't work"; negativity, in my view, speaks to the fact that life, in some sense, *doesn't* "work," is structurally inimical to happiness, stability, or regulated functioning, and that only the repetitive working through of what still doesn't work in the end—or works only until the radically non-relational erupts from within it once more—constitutes the condition in which something like flourishing could ever happen. For "flourishing," as I would use the term, refers neither to "happiness" nor to simple detachment from what doesn't work in life but rather to the effort to push beyond limits (internal and external both) imposed by the fantasy of the sovereign self (the self detached from negativity) or the optimism invested in happiness (as an end to the labor of trying to achieve it).

In any case, we both see sex as a site for experiencing this intensified encounter with what disorganizes accustomed ways of being. And as Lauren and I both want to suggest, that encounter, viewed as traumatic or not, remains bound to the nonfutural insistence in sex of something nonproductive, nonteleological, and divorced from meaning making. In this sense sex without optimism invokes the negativity of sex as a defining and even enabling condition. Gayle Rubin reminds us in "Thinking Sex" that "Western cultures generally consider sex to be a dangerous, destructive, negative force," to which we might add: if only sex lived up to such press more often

(Rubin 2011, 148)! If only, that is, the Panoptimism that rules us, even (or especially) in our denial of its hold, did not so often lend value to sex through the world-preserving meanings imposed upon it to repudiate its negativity. One need not romanticize sex to maintain that it offers, in its most intensely felt and therefore least routinized forms, something in excess of pleasure or happiness or the self-evidence of value. It takes us instead to a limit, and it is that limit, or the breaking beyond it, toward which sex without optimism points.

LB: I never suggested that flourishing involves a "simple" self-evidence in happiness that demands a detachment from "the bad life": flourishing involves traversing material conditions and then the affective sense of thriving, which is something different from and often incoherently bound to scenes and modes of living. This is why the materially "good life" might not be accompanied by a sense that life is good, why "good sex" might not be something one would want to repeat: without allowing for ambivalence, there is no flourishing. It therefore entails a complex navigation of life and noise, and the will to achieve it calls for practices and tendencies beyond mere accommodation to the world's and our own negativity. Likewise it isn't quite right to call psychoanalytic processes "structure" in *contrast* to the rule of misrule that marks ongoing modes of social domination: both domains of repetition structure, in that they are scenes in which subjects and scenes assume forms that have predictable, not determined, impacts. Structure is a process, not an imprint, of the reproduction of life.

De-antinomizing structure and the everyday, for example, one no longer has to see sex only as expressing a relation of power, or someone's singular pleasures, or the shattering activity of the drives. We wouldn't have needed Rubin to help us calm down and think about sex, and to think about affirming what's threatening about it either, if we did not need to figure out how sex reproduces normativity while predictably disorganizing assurance about why we want what we want and what our variety of attachments mean; at the same time, not quite knowing ourselves, we demand all sorts of things on behalf of the appetites, such as the right to anonymity, aggression, acknowledgment, pleasure, relief, protection, and, often, repair. Fantasy, formally speaking, is not what glosses over this craziness but that which makes it possible to move within it— sometimes in the blindingly glossy sense of optimism Lee proposes but more formally in the sense its setting provides that ambivalent, incoherent, proximate forces can be moved, moved through, and with. These processes of exposure to power, norm, and desire are structuring in their very variety and variation. As I wrote recently in an essay about the work of Leo Bersani and David Halperin, "When in a romance someone has sex and then says to the lover, 'You make me feel safe,' we understand that she means that there's been an emotional compensation to neutralize how unsafe and close to the abject sex makes her feel. 'You make me feel safe' means that I can relax and have fun where I am also not safe, where I am too close to the ridiculous, the disgusting, the merely weird, or—simply too close to having a desire. But some situations are riskier than others, as the meanings of unsafe sex change according to who's having the sex" (Berlant 2009, 266). That's where the politics comes in.

So when I say that I want to dedramatize our conceptual and embodied encounters with sex, I don't mean that I want to live in the pastoral sex world of *Shortbus* (Mitchell 2006), cruising like a happy puppy sniffing around a sea of interesting crotches. To some degree Lee is right that my stance is a way of making peace with misrecognition. Making peace with it, it seems to me—being a realist of sorts as well—gives us a shot at displacing sex from its normative function as the mechanism of emotional cohesion that sustains aggressive heteronormativity. But also, since misrecognition is inevitable, since the fantasmatic projection onto objects of desire that crack you open and give you back to yourself in a way about which you might feel many ways will always happen in any circuit of reciprocity with the world, why fight it? The question is where we move the dramatics of projection, what we can make available for changing their imaginary shape and consequence. I take cues from Lacan and Cavell to see sex as part of a comedy of misrecognition at the same time as it also can be a tragic drama of inflation and deflation. But "comedy" is a technical term here; it does not point to what's funny or what feels good. Comedy stages explosive and implosive problems of adjustment that are fundamentally affective and political— and survivable, if not affectively too bearable, even beyond the limit.

It might be worth mentioning this concept's origin in a high moment in feminist radicalism. I learned "dedramatize" first from reading Monique Wittig. In *The Straight Mind*, Wittig advocated dedramatizing gender (1992, 30). Her thought was that the demand to be intelligible as a gendered subject reproduced the prisonhouse of binary relationality that constantly reconstitutes heterosexuality as the norm on which all social intelligibility and standards of virtue are said to hang. I think, although I have never thought it before writing it here, that what motivates me to insist on a project of dedramatizing the very intense aim of remaining in attachment is not to deny the drama but to address it tenderly, nudging it to a new place the way a border collie would, not reproducing the intensity of the grand foundation for the world it has become, because only under those conditions of seeing dramas in their ordinariness will the virtue squad not be able to use dramas of threatened sexual security to reproduce the normative good life. To dedramatize the sexual encounter, to think of "benign variation" as sometimes really benign and not a disavowal of story's inevitable negativity, is to dedramatize disavowal and call it what it is, our partial understanding of what we're doing when we take up a position in proximity to the drives that bring us, once again, to becoming undone by wanting something, for example, by wanting sex.

This leads me to our archive. After all of this Lee and I looked at what we could possibly use to exemplify our views. He wants to think about the subject's radical negativity. I had thought I would want to show sex at the extremes, since no doubt the first definition of "sex without optimism" in the imaginary OED of the appetites would be bad sex, sex without pleasure, sex that was manifestly or tacitly coerced, forced, or compulsive, sex that disappoints or that turned out to be beside the point. But in my current scholarly work I am focusing on the nonmelodramatic affects that have come to saturate some sexually queer narratives, so that an optimistic structure might not sound like optimism at all—from the vocal flatness of memory films like *The Watermelon Woman, Chuck and Buck, Mysterious Skin*, and *My Life on Ice*, which tell a trauma story in the tonalities of indie coolness, to sexuality as a form of artifice or method acting in *Mulholland Drive* and *Boys Don't Cry*, to the affectively variable tender experimentality of adolescence films like *In Between Days*,

nerability without compulsively inducing a saturating defense that
attempts to disavow the noise of abandonment and dread.

What's Lost

LE: Loss is what, in the object-relation, it's impossible to lose; it's
what you're left with when an object changes its place or changes
its state. Even change for the better, even gain involves such loss,
where loss is not merely an emptiness but something more dimen-
sional, something that fills the vacated space that's left by what used
to be there. Loss, in such a context, may be a name for what survives. In the place of what one had before, loss remains to measure
the space or distance relation requires. As relationality's constant,
then, loss preserves relation in the absence of its object, affirming
the object's contingency, from which relation first takes its sting,
even if or when the object is mourned as irreplaceable. Maybe that's
one of the motives for Eve's engagement with reincarnation, with
the thought of surviving in and as this very *loss* of self, of *becoming*
that loss and maintaining thereby a relation that overcomes it.

At the end of "The Weather in Proust," for example, she quotes
this sentence from an account of Plotinus's thought on reincarnation: "When it passes from one inner level to another, the self
always has the impression that it is losing itself" (Sedgwick 2011,
34). But implicit here is a counterassertion: that such an impression
of the *loss* of self is something the self can *have*. Indeed that very impression may be what *constitutes* the self. Such a self would emerge
from the outset, through its experience of threatened loss, in the
paranoid position associated with what I've been calling the place
of the "no." What Eve evokes as the reparative position, anxiously
responding in its own distinct way to the anxiety of the paranoid,
would trope on this stance of negation by presenting the threat
as aimed at the object now instead of at the self, as emanating, in
fact, from *within* that self whose power—that is, whose *destructive*
power—fills the self with dread, but in doing so *fills the self* nonetheless.

Protecting, holding, pitying: the reparative process, as Eve asserts, may possess (unlike the schizoid position, with its murderous

assertiveness) a "mature, ethical dimension" (Sedgwick 2007, 638). "Among Klein's names for the reparative process," she tells us elsewhere, "is love" (Sedgwick 2003, 128). But that doesn't preclude reparativity's implication in violence, aggression, and destruction or exempt it from the consequences of its defensive deployment by a self whose dread of its powers nonetheless enlarges both them and it. And never more successfully than when that self would restrain or renounce them. This is the paradox of the reparative position and also, perhaps, of the mysticism Eve associates with reincarnation. For if mysticism in "The Weather in Proust" is, in Eve's words, "all but defined by its defiance of the closed system of either/or" then we might well ask, as the aural slippage between signifiers here suggests, if such defiance actually *defies* or *defines* what closes the system (Sedgwick 2011, 5). Doesn't the act of defiance perform the closed system's distinctive "no" and so reproduce the "either/or" it's intended to defy?

Closed or open: that is the question Eve's essay will force us to ask: "The important question in Proust" is "how open systems relate to closed ones, or perhaps better put, . . . how systems themselves move between functioning as open and closed" (Sedgwick 2011, 3). The "better" formulation's betterness, of course, depends on the greater openness seen in its invocation of *and*, but even that openness cannot close off the closed system's "either/or." We may now be asking how systems move "between functioning as open and closed," but the functions themselves, as "between" makes clear, remain resolutely digital, where the digital pertains to the paranoid position's insistence on saying "no." While that "no" by no means discredits mysticism's claims to potential openness (any more than the *and* as trope for *or* discredits reparativity), it betrays the negativity indissociable from every gesture of repair: the disjunction or "no" that registers loss as the medium of, the precondition for, and the spur to relationality.

LB: I don't know if *loss* is the best name for what survives, or what relation it has to your similar observation about failure. But I agree that what we're facing is a spectacle of an unspectacular space in Eve's work, of the subject's own capacity not to be caught up in the tangle of her own circuits of abjection, grandiosity, and aggression. What does it mean to be in them without being torn up by them? What is the relation of narrative contingency to her stated desire to be held, not through the will but by unconditional love? What does it mean to want to write relationality into the unconditional? More and more potential orientations toward the object proliferate. It is as though her pedagogical compulsion to make people smarter translates, after a while, into making them merely proximate, as in the intimate pedagogy she frames so magnificently in "White Glasses," where intimacy is about cospatiality and not predictability, recognition, or exchange. The unpredictable structure of the later work does not incite mourning in me or a desire to seduce the text toward repair but a curiosity about what's on offer in that space, a Bollasian attentiveness to the possibility of a loving deflation and a stretching out to figure things out, like a cat waking up in the sun. Perhaps the displacements she narrates are not always about loss and repair but a departure from the vanity of achieving perfect form and the risk of unlearning an attachment to the potential for drama to prove that we are really living.

This leads us back to dread: the dread of admitting knowing what brokenness is while managing the rage to repair. This living place of a knowing dread is a hard thing to talk about, much harder than the subject's tenderness, injury, and projected aggression. In some late-career moods Eve writes not in the emotional vernacular of empathy but with realism about how destructive pure being is:

> The Kleinian infant experiences a greed whose aggressive and envious component is already perceived as posing a terrible threat both to her desired objects and to herself. The resulting primary anxiety is an affect so toxic that it probably ought to be called, not anxiety, but dread. It is against this endogenous dread that the primary defense mechanisms are first mobilized—the splitting, the omnipotence, the violent projection and introjection. These defenses, in turn, which may be mitigated but never go away, can impress their shape on the internal experience of repression as well as the social experience of suffering from, enforcing, or resisting repression. (Sedgwick 2007, 633–34)

In this model, the subject who dreads is not successful at disavowal but spends her time encountering the impossible-to-distinguish relation between attaching and destroying and between building a world and annihilating what's inconvenient to it, including herself. Dread marks the core power of this version of the subject, no longer seen as protected by care and the compulsion to repair but as vulnerable to all acts, even acts of love, whose internal relation of violence to preservation is completely cloaked by the ambitions of personality to appear blameless.

LE: Listening to this powerful reading, Lauren, I'm conscious of the implicit drama you trace in the difficult gambit associated with Eve's "spectacle of [the] unspectacular"—a gambit perfectly captured when you write: "Perhaps the displacements [Eve] narrates are not always about loss and repair but [about] . . . the risk of unlearning an attachment to the potential for drama to prove that we are really living." That the real need not be situated in the inflated extremes of "drama" is surely a lesson that Eve learns through Klein (and through her therapist, Shannon, as well). But narratives evoking the "risk of unlearning" such histrionic attachments reenact them through the excitations called forth by the figure of "risk." Drama, like negativity, may be harder to escape than we think. Even the trope of "escaping" drama covertly resurrects it in the same way that self-enlargement may inhere in the effort to make the self minimal, to turn it from actor to witness, or to make such "witness" into something more companionate, more relational, like *withness*.

A middle child, as she lets us know in *A Dialogue on Love*, Eve bluntly acknowledges her profound distrust of melodramatic extremes, but she admits that the "middle ranges of agency" that allow for "negotiations" represent, at best, a "fragile achievement," always on the verge of coming undone and so bound up with dramatic suspense no less than with suspensions of drama. Eve, after all, loved the novel; she began her career with a book on the Gothic; and melodramatic extremes were sites of intense erotic potential. Yet she invests much in this space of detachment from the melodramatics of selfhood, invests, that is, in a holding environment as sustaining to us as air, as ubiquitous as weather: a space beyond grandiosity, splitting, anxiety, or dread, a space she lovingly specifies as "quotidian, unspecial, reality-grounded" (Sedgwick 2011, 4). But what relation obtains between such a space and the intensities of sex or the pressures of drives and desires that make that dread-free space so desirable?

Sometimes Eve posits that space of detachment as a vast circuit of interrelation. In *A Dialogue on Love* she describes it as "big / enough that you could never / even know whether // the system was closed, finally, or open" (Sedgwick 2000, 114). But if the openness of the system is open to doubt, the psychic affordance of this figure for interconnectedness is not; "picturing this new kind of circuitry was a vital *self-protective* step," she writes (115). Though for Eve the very point of this circuit "could only // lie in valuing / all the transformations and / transitivities // in all directions / for their difference" (114), that openness to transformation remains in the service of "self-protect[ion]," conserving what is, forestalling loss, and so precluding *her* transformation beyond a recognizable self insofar as she remains what sees and values the transformations around her. That is what becoming witness means here ("picturing this new kind of circuitry") and why witness, which Eve calls "reality-grounded," may not be so different from fantasy. Both rely on a loss of self through identification with the mise-en-scène in order to see what happens in what one imagines as one's absence. Eve distinguishes this open circuitry of what she calls "post-Proustian love" from the circulation of erotic desire in closed or triangular structures — structures in which

> you would
> eventually
>
> get back all of the
> erotic energy you'd
> sent around it (so
> that the point of this
> fantasy was *nothing is*
> *ever really lost)* —   (114)

But that fantasy continues to animate her thinking about reincarnation and mysticism. That, I think, is why Eve insists, by the time of "The Weather in Proust," that even a figure for reincarnation like the fountain of the Prince de Guermantes remains bound to the drama of a linear narrative, to a "conservation of matter and energy" that "might be called strictly karmic" (Sedgwick 2011, 3). And yet, as she notes, something other than the logic of karma is at play too, something that keeps the circuitry open to prevent the possibility that transformation, that novelty, might get lost. Observing how the fountain's elegant jets unexpectedly douse Mme d'Arpajon when a sudden gust of wind diverts them, Eve writes, "Sometimes things that come around don't go around, and vice versa" (3).

Beyond the cycles of karma, then, whether that karma turns out to be good or bad, reparative or paranoid, lies the space of "no karma" that every attempt to approach pushes farther away (just as seeking the space beyond drama, aspiring to inhabit its "beyond," already entails the *heroics* of drama in trying to supersede it). "It seems inevitable for us karmic individuals," Eve admits at the end of "Melanie Klein and the Difference Affect Makes," "that even the invocation of nonkarmic possibility will be karmically overdetermined. . . . It can function as an evasion" (Sedgwick 2007, 641–42). An evasion of the desire that attaches us to the vision of freedom from desire itself? An evasion of the historicity of our own relation to the "nonkarmic"? An evasion of the ways the nonkarmic may carry, as its very prefix suggests, the "no" that marks its connection to the splitting evinced by the schizoid position? Eve ends that essay without specifying just what the nonkarmic would evade, affirming instead that, at least for her, the "vision of nonkarmic possibility . . . also illuminates some possibilities of opening out new relations to the depressive position" (642).

Whatever this means, and I think Eve deliberately refuses to give us its meaning in any propositional form, it strikes the chord of a set of values to which the whole of her later work vibrates. "Possibilities," "opening out," "new relations": these sound the base tone of those values and they anticipate her explicit summation of them near the end of "The Weather in Proust": "That the universe along with the things in it are alive and therefore good: here I think is a crux of Proust's mysticism. Moreover, the formulation does not record a certainty or a belief but an orientation, the structure of a need, and a mode of perception. It is possible for the universe to be dead and worthless; but if it does not live, neither do the things in it, including oneself and one's own contents" (Sedgwick 2011, 32). The universe must live, and in living be good, these sentences seem to suggest, either *because* I am living myself or *in order that I may continue to do so*. Just before she makes this claim Eve talks about viewing the universe as "instinct with value and vitality" (32); here, in a parallel epithet, though one chiastically inverted, she recoils from seeing it as "dead and worthless." It's not just vitality that she values here, but value that proves to be vital: the *valuing* of the universe that sees it as good is precisely what keeps it alive.

The nonkarmic alternative to self-inflation brings us back to a self apparently charged with maintaining and supporting the universe *so that it can hold the self in turn*. As Eve muses in *A Dialogue on Love*, "Without magical thinking I imagine the world would be gray, no colors, air pushed out of it" (Sedgwick 2000, 111); this world without sequins, deprived of attachment, is the one and only thing, Eve tells us, she truly dreads for herself: "for me, dread only // I may stop knowing / how to like and desire / the world around me" (4). But the dread here attaches less to the prospect of detachment from the world, less to the specific thought of her neither liking nor desiring it, than to the competence-humbling confrontation with not "knowing how" to do so. An affective blockage gets processed as dread when its form is epistemological. Or else, as a defense against dread itself, epistemology here trumps affect. Of course, the tension between these two projects (epistemology and affect) names a rupture in Eve's career even as it names two competing ways in which she encounters Proust. Against what she acknowledges, but devalues, as his "demystifying, propositional level of knowingness and lack" (6) she mobilizes the nonkarmic alternative: "the non-propositional, environmental order of Proust's reality-orientation, which coincides with his mysticism" (Sedgwick 2011, 4). Between epistemology and object-relations, between the order of propositions and the environment they take place in, we encounter once more the place of the "no," the space of discontinuity, where knowingness, with its endless retinue of erotic potentiality bound up with the limit or lack that's always encountered in the "no," is deposed in favor of an ethical vitalization of the universe.

LB: I am not sure that being erotically knowing, in Eve's work, is trumped by a vitalizing ethical sanitation of the inconvenience and messiness of attachment. Is trumping the only relation we can see when divergent models line up next to each other? Are managerial impulses really, in the end, impulses toward mastery? These are not rhetorical questions, but I'm not saying yes or no. The transferential situation lets us encounter where we don't make sense without being defeated by it. I recognize that I read for what Eve makes possible, for her belief in the work of concepts to make the unbearable livable and the nonrelational part of intimacy a part of what's potentially sustaining in attachment. People often encounter their own dramas undramatically, with not much more than a nod and sometimes comic shrugging. Let me focus on a few related problems emerging in our analysis.

For Eve, dread opens up the possibility of seeing that one's own dramas are murderous and that this knowledge does not make them less murderous. What its acknowledgment does—and this is different from what knowledge does—is to specify those impulses as one mode of action among many. I could destroy the world in my dreaded desire for it—or not, and in the not, be rocked by things without being defeated by it. So at stake in the confrontation with the impulse to use knowledge and writing to repair a relationality constitutively broken while remaining relational is not to note that epistemology trumps affect or vice versa but to address how to proceed when one's epistemological and affective dressage no longer provides knowledge, pleasure, or even effective affect management. This is the conceptual rhetorical work of Eve's late fictocriticism, as well as the motive for therapy. The crisis is of what to do when one's long habit of doing the work of being oneself no longer works, not even in a fake or fantasmatic way: one needs all of one's resources for improvisation, new affective rhythms, better conceptualizations of what the subject is capable of that will always coexist with the aspect of the subject stuck in drama. Likewise, therefore, the problem in Eve's work of risking unlearning the association of life with a dramatics of living is not necessarily a fantasy of escape from drama but a fantasy of making room for the openness imminent to acknowledgment without destroying that space with the dreaded histrionics of one's greedy mastery demands.

Judging what is necessarily or not necessarily the case is a central trope throughout her work, and a trope is not necessarily a drama. It might involve feeling out a territory like a hand skipping over sand in the dark. When she says something "must necessarily" refer—as in "the nation must necessarily refer to sexuality"—it is to insist on the connectedness of things that claim to be separate, and it is always political (Sedgwick 1993, 147). But when the "not necessarily related" kind of phrase appears, it ratchets down the melodrama of attachment: "After this, in fact, I get very charmed and relaxed by everything that looks like non-necessity. I've started noticing that lots of Shannon's best comments—the ones that change the aspect of things for me—amount to nothing more profound than 'It ain't necessarily so'" (Sedgwick 2000, 112). One could call the discovery of the nonnecessity of things, a non- that's predicted by the spontaneity of the Sedgwickian nonce, a moment of heightening that also marks the difference between affect and emotion as vectors of analysis.

In the way she represents her relation to Shannon, Eve does sometimes wish for something simple, an emotional monotone that rules over the affectively inconvenient noise. This is because the noise of affect *is* inconvenient. But Eve was trying for something else in the work too—not a simple symptom simply calling out to be cured but a messier room. Symptoms overorganize a process into a representation. They seem literal: one problem, one presenting and representing problem. But before something becomes the lie that is a symptom, a fetish, or a fact invested with desire, it is a dispersed environment of causes and pulses. The unconscious is not where she looks to be able to bear this. She looks to her complex world made up of affective extensions. She calls Shannon, her friends, and the authors in whose work she is deeply invested forces that change the *aspect* of life, etymologically the arrangement of the planets, and she hopes that changing the aspect can change the expect. The question is whether the wish to provide a rearrangement is a defense against the loss of everything or a wish for the unbearable to become the habitable in a way that actually risks changing something. My gamble is that the encounter with her unconditional negativity, the misalignment of her internal planets, is not the same thing as merely a fantasy of being both oneself and otherwise. It matters to say "maybe." Acknowledgment changes a palate.

This takes me directly to sex. *A Dialogue on Love* narrates the loss of a lifelong masturbatory practice and its refinding as erotic energy both in the transferential therapeutic scene and outside the office as well: just as the "dialogue" on love is not a dialogue but many genres of call and response, so too she finds sex again in anything that can stand as a syncopated relation. Syncopation includes syncope, a fainting feeling. She finds it all, the recession and the return, in caring for the other, in being cared for, in allowing the other to push her body into a new aspect and make it feel solid and liquid; in the concept of a being-with that includes all of what's unshared and discarded in the penumbra of the promise to show up again for more talk; and in the revelation that there was never a singular break to be repaired but tears within a membrane that can take the shock in some spots better than others, without being annihilated by it.

In this way out-of-synchness is not only a drama of negativity but also sociality's great promise, and a way to maintain an affective mess for which most people do not have the skill or the trust in the world's, or other people's, patience. Eve never wrote an essay called "Pedagogy of Sex." There are many reasons for this, no doubt, and "A Poem Is Being Written" comes close. There the main thing is that sex is not a thing of truth but a scene where one discovers potentiality in the abandon that's on the other side of abandonment. She wanted sex at once to expand and become specific by multiplying the range of its potential scenarios and relational rhythms, so that her readers, her intimates could achieve different kinds of aspect-altering acknowledgment of sexuality's genuinely wild object inducements, from the biggest love to something as minimal as a "gay-affirmative detachment" (Sedgwick 1993, 169).

So I am not saying to you, "Stop with all the drama, already!" Sometimes Eve said things like that, but it was just one of her many wishes. Others were to acknowledge the subject's internal chaos in relation to the chaos of the world; to admit the relief of being managed and managing the situation of attachment without repairing it, were repairing to mean disavowal; and to imagine that different tones could induce unpredicted infrastructures for relationality in the world. Above all, to respect the impact of the concept a wish makes to reroute the effects, and the affects.

LE: I'm glad you're not saying "Stop with all the drama, already!" since such a self-deconstructing imperative would be a showstopper in spite of itself. We could hardly stop the drama, after all, and still produce a dialogue. Whether delivering this talk at the MLA in a give-and-take always alive to the fear of annihilation through a "zinger," intended as such or not, or here in the space of the printed page where our separate but interwoven words still function contrapuntally, we're mired to our eyeballs in drama—the drama we've known since Plato inheres in encountering an idea but that also inheres, as we've known since Sigmund Freud, in the negativity of relation. The question is how we stage that drama, both for others and for ourselves, and how it stages us.

Together and separate, Lauren and Lee: bound by the dialogic structure that also distinguishes our voices, we're certain to be staged, whether we like it or not, as instantiating the hendiadic logic of "Paranoid Reading and Reparative Reading." Not that you and I occupy, as if we were allegorical figures, the reparative and paranoid positions respectively (or as if those positions themselves, as I've been arguing, are ever as clear-cut as they seem), but we're certainly susceptible to misrecognition in those binarizing terms. Though we share, that is, a resistance to the pastoral affirmation of cohesiveness, though we both see Eve herself as producing something beyond the repair that endlessly animates rupture's "no," we nonetheless, and perhaps unavoidably given the form in which we're working, subject ourselves to the risk of construction in allegorical terms. Viewed through the distortion of such a lens, I would embody the negativity Eve distrusts in paranoia: the negativity she associates with the demystications practiced by the Yale school, whose "masculine" regime of epistemological power she opposes to "vitality and value" and so to the prospect of aesthetic coherence imagined as "weather" or "environment."

That same false optic would identify you with the affect theory through which Eve envisions an access to immediacy, to the plenitude of possibility, to a less anxious relation to the body, and to a nondestructive, nondualistic ability to be with what is. As understood in this way by Eve, affect theory permits movement beyond the ruptures resurrected by repair, even if only in ways that one— or at least the allegorical *other* one who figures paranoid reading— might describe as largely enacting a fantasmatic repair *of* repair. Affect theory, as Eve conceives it, which is not, as we know, how you do, envisions the possibility of a universe of good: a holding environment that opens a space beyond histrionic extremes and the lethal conflicts of either/or. That version of affect theory, by holding on to the possibility of the subject's being held (hence neither abandoned nor allowed to drop), occupies the fantasmatic place of the good, or the good enough, mother for Eve, whether that mother be identified with Shannon or with the text of À la recherche. And though such a version of affect theory differs markedly from yours, our audience, Lauren, may align you too with Eve's conflation of affect theory and a sustaining maternal hold. Not because you believe in that hold as what affect theory offers, but because Eve, in enlisting affect to affirm the prospect of repaired relation, of the openness of and to "being with," employs your language to imagine a dread-free coexistence with mess. She reads the potentiality inherent in weather—in a quotidian, "reality-grounded" environment—as what holds us by holding out to us the promise of "value and vitality," of the universe as a livable space.

If you face allegorical inscription, though, in the place of the good enough mother, then I, like the paranoid practices of deconstructive knowingness, am likely to be cast, and no less falsely (at least from my point of view), as theory's equivalent of Darth Vader, a form of the father we love to hate: withholding, histrionic, life-negating, and full of inhuman enjoyment. In such an allegorical setup, though, where both of us get set up (and not by reason of gender alone, though gender will play a role), I'm made to figure something Eve resolutely sought to project, while you figure something Eve equally resolutely wanted to incorporate. And just as neither you nor I conform to these allegorical images (though saying so won't forestall in the least our assimilation to them), so Eve, or the Eve that survives as her texts, is distinct from the self that such acts of projection and incorporation would induce. Her texts show those acts, or perhaps we should define them as *tendencies* instead, to be wishes, desires, karmic strivings bound up with the drama of trying to overcome her own intractable resistance. You write, and for me quite movingly, "I read for what Eve makes possible"; I, on the other hand, read in Eve's text what makes its coherence *impossible*. You resonate to what you call Eve's "belief in the work of concepts to make the unbearable livable and the nonrelational part of intimacy a part of what's potentially sustaining in attachment," while I respond to her text's incapacity to resolve into such propositional utterances without, in the end, repudiating the very privilege of propositional thought.

I view as serious reflections on the different ways we read the series of questions you generate in response to my take on Eve's work: "Is trumping the only relation we can see when divergent models line up next to each other? Are managerial impulses really, in the end, impulses toward mastery?" No doubt there are other models than trumping for thinking what happens when antithetical constructs appear beside each other. But as the contexts of our readings must count for something, so must the language Eve uses. When *A Dialogue on Love* first broaches dread, the book's most troubling affect (and most troubling precisely insofar as it springs from the prospect of love's undoing), she locates it, where dread *for herself* is concerned, *uniquely* in a failure of *knowing*—specifically a failure of *knowing how* to mobilize attachment to the world. In that sense the failure of knowledge, I argued, might be the form, however displaced, that affective blockage takes. Or it might, alternatively, function defensively to trump the incursion of affect. For me, then, the question is not whether trumping is "the only relation we can see when antithetical models line up," but why *in this instance*, when she first explores dread, Eve focuses explicitly on epistemological failure; why the impulse to affect that's figured by dread of a lost attachment to the world takes the form of what affect in Eve would displace: the insistence of epistemological mastery. I'm not interested in globalizing this particular move and making such mastery the secret desire of Eve's writings, both early and late. I want to focus instead on the negativity inseparable from her career-long pursuit of a survivable self—the negativity implicit in her trying and failing to cast out paranoia while also trying and failing to incorporate what affect theory might promise. But "failing," in Eve's case as much as in ours, fails as a name for this practice; for her, too, the want that compels repetition is just what relation most wants.

This repetition has much to do with both survival and affect management. Wanting to allow for what you hail as "sociality's great promise," wanting to provide a space for what you describe as "affective mess," and so for living with an incoherence that needn't prove to be murderous, you ask if "managerial impulses" must, in the end, aspire to mastery. But precisely as an effort to evade the murderousness of paranoid-schizoid splitting, affect management, at least in Eve's work, does aim to master a threat. And that threat is itself an affect: the dread Eve traces to a failure of knowledge.

To make a very long argument short, the discourse of affect management for Eve seems to function like, but as an alternative to, the Freudian reality principle. Hence she characterizes affect theory as thoroughly grounded in reality. She writes, for example:

> [Melanie Klein's] work has a reassuring groundedness, a sense of reality. I realize that this remark may sound implausible to anyone willing to sail through sentences about the cannibalistic defense of the good partial breast against the devouring invasion of the feces. But . . . I feel enabled by the way that even abstruse Kleinian work remains so susceptible to a gut check. It may not be grounded in common sense, but it is phenomenologically grounded to a remarkable degree. A lot of this quality is owing to the fact that Klein's psychoanalysis, by contrast to Freud's, is based in affect. (Sedgwick 2007, 628)

The capacity to tolerate disturbance, to put up with frustration undramatically, to be with and amid contradiction without resorting to murderous violence: that's what the reality principle affords, and that's why, for Freud, the reality principle and the pleasure principle aren't antithetical; instead the former temporalizes the latter in the service of survival. In this nonopposition the reality principle registers and manages affect by binding the otherwise freely mobile energy of the primary process. This reality-based affect management aims for an overall feeling of evenness as a version of pleasure that's more stable, modulated, and controlled than the primary process's. This may explain why Eve takes great pains to link affect theory's grounding in "reality," and hence its attention to the possibilities for "respond[ing] to environmental (e.g., political) change" (Sedgwick 2003, 144), with the reparative's investment in pleasure (as opposed to paranoia's investment in knowledge): "Reparative motives, once they become explicit, are inadmissible in paranoid theory both because they are about pleasure . . . and because they are frankly ameliorative" (144). Her recourse to a version of affect theory thus brings reality and pleasure together, and this pairing sketches the outlines of a nonkarmic alternative to paranoia.

But beyond the reality and the pleasure principles lies the death drive's repetitions—the pressure of a negativity that insists as a surplus of form over content, of structure over statement, of performance over meaning. Though Eve wanted something other than the death drive's otherness to life, that wanting preserved the place in which its otherness survived. What her work, with its restless intelligence and unyielding commitment asks of us, and what we, in being true to it, have been asking of each other, is whether the *and* can embrace the *or* without, in the process, repeating *or*'s own otherness to *and*. Does such an embrace, in other words, depend on the distance it would abrogate and the negativity it would deny? Which also may be a way of asking: In such an embrace, what survives?

LB: We converge in seeing that reparativity, in Eve's work, marks the and/or in an insuperable negativity that induces nonetheless a wish for relief in repair, which may mean something as minor but major as a shift in attachment styles. But, at the same time, I would argue that the very shifting of the subject in response to its own threat to its self-attachment can be the source of an affective creativity that is not just a fantasmatic toupée, but also the possibility of a recalibrated sensorium, as when a comic orientation toward aggression and pleasure produces new capacities for bearing, and not repairing, ambivalence. Eve's work is a training in being in the room with that ambivalence, which she also called unbearable, in its revelation that having and losing are indistinguishable; although sometimes, for example, while one is mourning, it does not feel that way.

3. LIVING WITH NEGATIVITY

LEE EDELMAN: We've been thinking about sex in relation to negativity and politics in order to reassert its importance at a moment
when much of contemporary critical thought (and much of contemporary activist practice) seems, in our view, all too eager to put the
subject of sex behind it. Critical discourse now centers instead on
questions of rights (civil, natural, and human), of sovereign power
and states of exception, of the definition and limits of the human,
and of the distribution and control of populations through the categories of citizen and noncitizen. Sex, in this context, can carry the
odor of anachronism, narcissism, or something irreducibly and dis-
concertingly personal, and any impulse to linger on its place in the
social, cultural, and political fields can suggest a stubbornly narrow
gaze or a refusal to move on.

To be sure, this makes a certain sense insofar as sex can be said
to resist such narratives of moving on, naming instead the site
where desire, for all its potential mobility, remains fixed to a primal
attachment that alone makes our objects appear as desirable. The
movement produced by this combination of mobility and attachment defines, at least in Lacanian terms, the circuit of the drive in
its orbit around an inaccessible (non)object (what Lacan calls the
objet a) whose gravitational pull is reflected in the series of objects
metonymically invested with desire that would take that (non)ob-
ject's place. Insofar as this leaves the subject torn between desire as
a form of representation (of the *objet a* that cannot be objectified)
and the unrepresentable cause of desire that attaches us to attachment itself, it speaks to the negativity of sex, to our nonsovereign
status as subjects. What we know of ourselves as desiring subjects

remains fixed, that is, to the unknowable frame in which all such knowing occurs—fixed to the particular libidinal structure that enables but also disrupts it. The calculations by which the desiring subject attempts to take its own measure are thrown off, therefore, by the unknown attachments that determine the measure it chooses. Though the subject endeavors to routinize this being out of joint with itself—to inhabit its environment, as Eve might put it—some experiences intensify the pressure of that disjunctiveness or incoherence, insisting on the negativity that structures the drive's relation to desire.

With this as our context, I want to begin by returning to something that Lauren pointed out in chapter 1: "We both see sex as a site for experiencing this intensified encounter with what disorganizes accustomed ways of being," and we both proceed from a recognition of "the subject's constitution by and attachment to varieties of being undone." But that undoing has different consequences in Lauren's work and in mine, largely because we read it from different, though clearly related perspectives. For Lauren, the impulse to historicize—and by doing so, to particularize—how different subjects differently experience the sense of their encounters with undoing reflects her more phenomenological investment in theorizing ways of negotiating and managing such disorganizations of being. She's committed, like Eve, to the political project of imagining and making possible a relation to the world not shadowed by threat or the defensive dramatization of differences as existential dangers. She proposes instead that we attend to the possibility of "making peace with" or "being in the room with" what she calls the "mess" of affective intensities by engaging that mess in its ordinariness instead of as inherently traumatic. What she calls her "utopian" aspect inheres in this belief that the conditions supporting abjection, aggression, and domination by norms are susceptible to transformation in ways that won't dramatize their negativity by defensively disavowing that negativity but might enable us, instead, to accept it as part of our openness to the world. Difference, conceived as "benign variation," might thus give rise to a vitalizing experience of engagement and curiosity rather than encouraging a fearful retreat to normativity's fortified bunkers. In this way she elaborates a transformative politics rooted in a commitment to the optimism by which we "stay bound to the world" and thus to its possibilities for undoing and rerouting our genres of attachment themselves.

Focusing instead on structures that insist through historical variation, I see undoing less as the subject's incoherence in the face of normativity than as the momentary access to a sense of its radical unrepresentability. Such negative encounters, such ruptures in the logic—which is always a *fantasy* logic—by which the subject's objects (itself included) yield a sense of the world's continuity (even if only the continuity of experiencing the world as incoherent), impose the abruptions that Lauren calls drama and undertakes to dedramatize. But in my understanding of how attachment binds the subject to the world, a tear in the fabric of attachment, and so in reality's representation, cannot be separated from threat or from the dramatics of undoing. The suggestion that heteronormative reproductions of the "good life" might be interrupted by dedramatizing the experience of rupture and "seeing dramas in their ordinariness" presupposes, in the very recognition of and attachment to ordinariness, the consistency that the subject is trying to achieve by dedramatizing in the first place. The subject, that is, so positioned to "see" its drama as ordinariness is not encountering the sort of undoing with which I'm most concerned.

Managing affective intensities by recognizing their status as part of the ordinary puts the emphasis on a cognitive binding of the subject to the world of its representations—the very binding under pressure of undoing in the encounters to which I refer. Such transformative self-perception achieved amid affective discontinuity implicitly presumes a mastery of, and a capacity to include in our calculations, our unknowable primal attachments. In this it risks a regression from engaging the nonsovereignty of the subject. At the same time, rather than obviating the subject's experience of threat, it displaces the threat of undoing onto the subject of dedramatized "seeing," a subject still defensively invested in the continuity of its representations precisely insofar as its incoherence is stabilized *by being seen as ordinary*—a stabilization whose reassurance can look like what social norms afford.

In "Sex without Optimism" Lauren and I began our approach to negativity while mapping our shared perspectives and the points at which they diverge; we examined negativity's relations to drama and disavowal in "What Survives," thinking in particular about ruptures in attachment and fantasies of repair. But a question Lauren raised at the outset still remains largely unanswered and might be taken as the impetus to our conversation here. "Since misrecognition is inevitable," Lauren wrote, "since the fantasmatic projection onto objects of desire that crack you open and give you back to yourself in a way about which you might feel many ways will always happen in any circuit of reciprocity with the world, why fight it?" This question rightly confronts my own description of negativity with the need to address the political consequences of its structural account of the subject. If attachment to the framework of representation defines the social subject, then what are the alternatives to the misrecognitions that at once domesticate the unknowable and consolidate the subject of representation? What politics proceeds from undoing, from breakdowns in the subject's forms of attachment? What would it mean, from within the context of our approaches to undoing, to take seriously the question of what it means to face living with negativity?

LAUREN BERLANT: In love, in collaboration, in ordinary interaction, and in scenes of potential attunement like teaching or theorizing, the impossibility of getting the account precisely right—even if one says plausible words and even if the interlocutor mainly concurs—often requires a tacit agreement not to push too hard on the object organizing the interaction. Here the object is the encounter between negativity and nonsovereignty, the problems of radical incoherence and relational out-of-synchness that threateningly traverse the subject and the world. So it surprises me not at all that Lee's representation of my relation to negativity makes me feel pedantic and also makes me laugh at my own will to tweak this chapter's opening, for that very will to will accuracy—to make what I might call "the misrecognition we can bear"—makes up the consistency of relationality as such, the texture that emerges from adjusting representations across the intimate and the political.

For the record, I have not actually been advocating a mode of reparative openness that "replaces" nonsovereignty, nor seeking one not "shadowed" by it. I am not trying to separate anything out from threat or "the dramatics of undoing," nor looking for a neutralizing repair. I don't deny the drama of what's unbearable in one's own negativity, but I do not think that drama has to feel dramatic or that, however it manifests, its appearance evidences the same "fact" of negativity regardless of context. I am arguing that it matters that and how we acknowledge both our affective discomposure in relation and the forms of misrecognition we improvise in ongoing negotiation with the sense of it, for those forms change how we encounter the intractable antagonisms and incoherences. Proposing to induce different settings from within a dynamic so as to change the becoming-form of an encounter—what I would call "politics" but which could also be called "aesthetics"—is not the same as substituting a new, better structure for an old, bad one. The affective event is not external to the structure but part of it too. Thus I am not claiming that normativity, hetero or otherwise, induces nonsovereignty *as opposed to* the threat to the subject's ontological disorganization. I am saying that both politics and pedagogy emerge from within the disturbing encounter of these various modes of being incomplete, contradictory, and out of control. Nonsovereignty can engender different atmospheres and potentials, and the structures of self-discontinuity and the place of fantasy in shifting, remediating, and revisceralizing its threat are more than extraneous noise and variation, are not always only failed attempts at adequation or mastery, and are where all kinds of significant transformations happen. So if Lee is tracking "structures that insist through historical variation," I am feeling out a different understanding of structure and a more integrated understanding of structure and fantasy— to what in these chapters I have called, variously, noise, variation, and tweaking—at the scene of living with our self-misrecognition. Negativity, like all objects, avails us a threat, an anchor, and the constant presence of failure and optimism. Whether or not all of this pressure produces futile gestures toward "mastery," for me it also offers the possibility of significant affective transformation— which is to say, a transfigured relation of drama to dramatics— which I take to be the source of its fundamentally political import. It matters that I could have written none of this without the working through and debating of the previous two chapters; I've learned a lot from this conversation.

Lee and I turned to this chapter to induce a development in the positioning we've elaborated in the previous two dialogues with respect to bearing the unbearable encounter with the unfinished business of being—not just its incompleteness but also in its desire for and resistance to being accounted for. As Lee has suggested, the earlier chapters address sex as a scene for staging the structural nonsovereignty of the subject and its relation to perturbed and incoherent relationality in the world, and we are looking also to the modes of threat that the world engenders and their inseparability from relations of love and attachment. Hence there are many scenes of "the political." Each operation involves the relief in fantasy, an anchoring to a sense near representation that provides some confidence in the endurance of the world and one's movement through it. To the extent that this chapter is about narrative and the encounter, then, to me this chapter is also about fantasy, including the fantasy of theory and its relation to how narrative binds and seduces us toward impossible repairs and resolutions.

So we have turned, as our anchor, to a story about an attempt to get an account of something right. We will be converging on Lydia Davis's "Break It Down," a story manifestly about accounting for relationality. We include it as an appendix to this volume so that there will be something outside of the hermeticism of the idiom we develop between us for debating living with negativity. Using it as our common resource, we will be asking whether and how it matters to respond to the problem of living with negativity, with its own radical self-incoherence and incommensurability, and we will ask whether "mastery" and "disavowal" are adequate names for what comes next, as we move within our encounter not only with our inevitably traumatic nonsovereignty but also the unruliness of the world. All page references for extracts from Davis's "Break It Down" refer to the reprinted story in the appendix to this volume.

LE: If dialogue continuously affords us new occasions to feel ourselves misrecognized, as Lauren cogently notes, that's in part because the unspoken desire by which conversation is sustained can turn imprecisions into misrepresentations as grossly disfiguring as a funhouse mirror, but without the surcharge of fun. To encounter another is to have to confront our otherness to ourselves. The wonder is not that we get things wrong; dialogue tends to proceed, after all, as much by identifying and correcting misreadings as by concurring with the other's account. No, the wonder is that the micro-abrasions that tear the relational filament are precisely what, in certain circumstances, serve to make it stronger, much as a muscle develops through the repetition of stress. Where negativity, encounter, and dialogue are concerned, we might remember the words of William Blake from *The Marriage of Heaven and Hell*: "Opposition is True Friendship" (Blake 2008, 42). Or, as I might rephrase the proverb to fit the current context: Thinking With and Against are the Same.

The encounter performed by this dialogue centers on the question of encounter as such: how to live relationality; how to confront our self-division; how to experience the unbearable undoing of the logic that binds us to the world; how to share a thought or an object when the pressure of its handling by another risks breaking the object, our willingness to share it, or our ability to cathect it. The question of encounter compels us to ask how the negativity of the subject's nonsovereignty, and so the division that makes us, simultaneously, the (conscious) subjects of our statements and the (unconscious) subjects of their enunciation, can still yield forms of relation sustaining both intimate and political bonds. Can the primary process as site of undoing, of implacable resistance to the binding of energy in stable representations, leave room nonetheless for living with negativity in ways that don't just shore up the ego for our survival or self-defense?

This question, frequently asked of my work on queer theory and the death drive, demands that we think more closely the join between the psychic and the social, between sex as the incoherence produced by the drive's irreducible otherness and experience as organized with regard to the broadly political fictions of sovereignty. Where Lauren affirms "the possibility of significant affective transformation" and sees in this "transformed relation of drama to dramatics" the "source" of her thinking's "fundamentally political import," I maintain that political import inheres no less in asserting the structural constraints on such transformation, the constraints that political discourse routinely promises to overcome. But it's not a matter of choosing one side and repudiating the other, even if that assertion ("it's not") repeats the insistence on repudiation that its statement disavows (much like the claim about mysticism's "defiance of the closed system of either/or" [Sedgwick 2011, 5]). What Wallace Stevens (1954/1990, 403) describes as "not a choice between / But of" remains, despite that description, a choice between *between* and *of*; it's just that choosing *of* requires the choice of *between* as well (and with it the exclusional force of *between* that *of* must now include). In the negativity essential to critical thought, thinking with and against are the same. Thus Lauren's utopianism fully acknowledges the persistence of structural constraints even as my focus on what's intractable in negativity wagers that the encounter with its queerness can change how we think and live the political.

But how does the queer negativity of the drive fit together with political thought? Teresa de Lauretis has brilliantly argued for their radical incommensurability, associating the former (particularly in my work) with rhetoric, irony, and figuration and the latter with the "fact-based" literality that the reality principle demands. The problem, she notes, resides in the difficulty of translation from one to the other insofar as "self-reflexive irony . . . is incompatible with the business of politics, as are all rhetorical figures that fissure the solidity of meaning" (de Lauretis 2011, 257). But to the extent that such solidity itself is no more than a rhetorical effect, taking shape as the irony of a figural practice whose counterpart is fantasy (the fantasy, that is, of an object to stabilize the dissolutions effected by irony), politics already bears within it the pressure of the drive. The literality, that is, to which politics appeals already bespeaks an irony—the very irony that enables politics, as the negativity of dissent, continuously to dispute and dissolve any putative "solidity of meaning." Far from being at odds with the fissures that irony occasions, politics performs the ceaseless, evental eruption of irony itself (where irony expresses the nonsovereignty we encounter in our status as subjects of language). In that case politics might be redescribed outside its insistent teleological imperatives and future-oriented acts. It might be seen, that is, as the insistence of a structural antagonism that undoes the totalization of meaning to which it seems to aspire. "A *political* community," to quote Jacques Rancière, "is in effect a community that is structurally divided, not between divergent interest groups and opinions, but divided in relation to itself" (Rancière, 115). That division, which politics opens through its dissensus from the social count, through "its supplementary symbolization in relation to any counting of the population and its parts" (115), suggests that the "fissure in the solidity of meaning," far from being, as de Lauretis hypothesizes, "incompatible with the business of politics," may actually define it. Or define, at least, the formal conflict intrinsic to this notion of politics as the drive-like oscillation between the "solidity of meaning" it seems to enunciate and the act of enunciation itself as the renewal of social division.

De Lauretis is right to associate politics with the construction of literality, but literality, as Lacan reminds us, is, etymologically, the figure of a letter: "But how are we to take the letter here? Quite simply, literally" (1966/2006, 413). Such a letter, as Lacan goes on to note, can produce "all its truth effects in man without the spirit having to intervene at all" (424). How, then, can we think the political relation, or the politics of relationality, without also thinking about the figural movements that produce it as object of thought and the literalization that tries to obscure all trace of that figural origin? Is politics the fantasy, when you break it down, of breaking down figures of fantasy? And if sex, as we've argued, can be seen as a name for what breaks down the fantasy of sovereignty, does it speak to the breaks and breakings down that go by the name of politics? As we turn to Lydia Davis's story, trying to share it and to break it down without breaking the relational thread that binds us to each other and to the object, we find ourselves facing the demand, once again, to think both with and against.

LB: As with sex and politics, theory is that to which we look both to disturb things and to repair them. But Lee and I begin with problems that are not reparable by theory or, perhaps, by anything. So the questions that we pose are really statements about a problem, not calls for a tucking in of the question. But there are always defenses against the play of encounter. As in politics and sex, in theory the encounter induces all the concomitant dread and excitement at the potential for something to become different.

The negativity with which Lee moves is the place where social and political antagonisms match the contours of the singular subject's incapacity to bear his internal divisions. But then, also, as political antagonisms are only "drive-*like*" and not an extension of the drive's own divisiveness, the question becomes what relation political nonsovereignty has to fantasy, and how that relation articulates with the subject's encounter with her internally chaotic tendencies. Are political and sexual fantasy the same structure thematically varied? What is the relation of unconscious fantasy to narrated and projected fantasies, since both enable ways of being in the world and involve struggling to corral symbols into a set that makes sense (in personality, the biography of being reliable, or as ideology)?

This question of structure's relation to representation, noise, or variation is why we turn to "Break It Down" to break down the broken relation we call negativity. "Break It Down" involves an unnamed narrator trying to break down an overwhelming emotional event by detailing the different kinds of investment he has made in a brief erotic encounter, investments financial, temporal, affective, and now memorial. It is a detailing whose desperation emerges clearly because the protagonist has none of the couple form's normative noise inside of which to hide his calculations for love. How does any account of subjectivity deal adequately with the affective and gestural aspects of being in relation when the inconvenience of the other who is both oneself *and* the others near oneself (actually and psychically) threatens thriving in common, while relation nonetheless goes on anyway? What does it mean to bring a language of accounting to a place surpassing accountability?

In some ways "Break It Down" is a story about trying to anchor an account of relationality to *pronouns*: a narrator's "I" is listening to a "he" who tells a story as "I" but then switches between "I" and "you" as he generalizes his processing of his love object, as he makes their relation into a case study of relationality itself. Meanwhile the beloved "her" who is a "she" in his recounting is a singular figure who comes to stand in for anything lost—even in the ordinary sense in which the biographical subject is lost, in a pronoun. Her imminent loss of physical presence is confirmed at the very end by a shirt that she gives him. The gifting of the shirt is impulsive— "gifting" might be too strong a word. And, as in all collaboration, any impulse to transfer an intimate object between intimates produces a scene both shared and unshared. Perhaps the impulse to give the intimate other a thing is in many genres of forcing, bullying, gifting, giving, inciting, sharing, refusal, presence, penance, dissociation, and so on.

> Another bad time, or it wasn't exactly bad, but it wasn't easy either, was when I had to leave, the time was coming, and I was beginning to tremble and feel empty, nothing in the middle of me, nothing inside, and nothing to hold me up on my legs, and then it came, everything was ready, and I had to go, and so it was just a kiss, a quick one, as though we were afraid of what might happen after a kiss, and she was almost wild then, she reached up to a hook by the door and took an old shirt, a green and blue shirt from the hook, and put it in my arms, for me to take away, the soft cloth was full of her smell. (Break It Down, 132)

Imminent to departing he takes the shirt of the woman whom he will no longer see and immediately begins to smell for her on the shirt. At that moment she might as well have disappeared, as she has provided a transitional object to stop the plot, the plotting for kisses that Adam Phillips argues is a fundamental narrative drive of the subject on discovering her constitutive aloneness (1993). On the other side of plotting for kisses, there is being in loss. Smelling a shirt is a thing people do with the intimate dead, the dead-to-me kind as well as the biologically departed: they smell the remaining clothing until the trace of the person has decayed beyond the nose's capacity to retrieve it. Sometimes this is not a matter of choice; the loved one's odor generates an atmosphere that must be breathed, that persists beyond cleanings. As the second skin of the soon departed, the experientially dead, the no longer physically present, the shirt represents the space of apostrophe that any intimacy involves, externalizing the internal distances that one makes so as not to be overwhelmed by the overpresence embodied even on the ordinarily near horizon. Only once the other has been even a little vanquished is she available to be loved.

But at the moment of absolute departure, the internally distancing defenses that make relation possible disappear, and the result is that the second narrator becomes a man without an infrastructure, a mess, "nothing in the middle of me, nothing inside, and nothing to hold me up on my legs." I am so interested in the literalization of nonsovereignty, the unwanted ideation and virtually skeletal dissolution that scenes of desire induce as pleasure, terror, and confusion. The narrative tracks him in this gesture, at a transitional moment to which he feels physically unable to navigate an adaptation, by handing him the shirt. The shirt returns him to his skeleton, which is not to say that it returns him to an identity that represses his ambivalence, his confusion, or his awareness that the relation floats on an enigma that cannot be too disturbed if contact is to endure. A skeleton is a framework for what makes living on possible. The shirt is a skin that demands a skeleton, that here brings it into being, pointing to a plan for action. There would be no narrative retrospect without the shirt. But it is not as though the act or its narration diminishes the mess of the narrator's sensorium. Both events organize and disorganize; they redistribute nonsovereignty and open relationality within the manifolds of the negativity within the attachment scene.

Of course there is much more to say. How do you read this gesture, at the last moment of their exchange?

LE: In beginning to read this object to which you've asked me to respond (where the "object" is not only the "gift" of the shirt but also your account of it), I'm struck by your insight in framing us—as collaborators and intimates—within the logic of exchange that Davis's text explicitly engages. Can I take the object you pass on to me, redolent as it is of your intellectual touch, and recognize, in your analysis, what I saw in "Break It Down"? Is the object in this shared encounter the same, or do its contours change on account of attachments, including some unaccounted for, that condition our accounts? Does accounting itself presuppose the fantasy of an Other who guarantees our math by seeing what we leave out? These questions are central to "Break It Down" and to the forms of relation that it, and we, want to think in terms of sex.

For whatever else the story does, it parses the problem of defining an encounter—of determining whether or not it takes place and of knowing precisely in what it consists—by reducing it first to a finite number of delimited sexual acts. When the man attempting to price the time that he spent with his female companion starts "breaking it all down," he first tallies the expenses incurred in the course of the ten days they enjoyed together (which he estimates at $1,000) and divides that amount by what he perceives as the goods he received in return: "And we made love, say, once a day on the average. That's $100 a shot. And each time it lasted maybe two or three hours so that would be anywhere from $33 to $50 an hour, which is expensive" (127). But the ratio of cost to benefit changes as the man continues his reflections and determines that more and more time should be added to his reckoning of what he calls "[the] time it lasted." The self-contained units of value he begins with, instances of "ma[king] love" quantifiable at "$100 a shot," expand to encompass more various aspects of the man's affective experience as he meditates on just what counts as part of the "sexual encounter."

What strikes me as most important here reinforces your keen observation about the story's attempt "to anchor an account of relationality to *pronouns*." But where your reading focuses on the distribution of subjects as, variously, "I," "you," "he," and "she," mine sees the central pronoun as one your account doesn't mention: "it." The title of the story, from this perspective, could just as well be "Break 'It' Down" since "it" and its variants, "its" and "it's," make over 120 appearances in the brief eight pages of the tale. More than just a matter of quantity (even if the narrative occasions such mimetic calculations as my own), the centrality of "it" to the story lies in our and the speaker's inability to know or specify what "it" is. Breaking "it" down enlarges it, changing our sense of the object itself. With his first assertion, "I'm breaking it all down," the man seems secure in his ability to circumscribe, define, and comprehend "it" (127). "It lasted maybe two or three hours" at a time, he announces near the outset, where "it" here refers to each act of lovemaking in its itemized particularity. Like Davis's later story, "How It Is Done," "Break It Down" seems to correlate "it" with sex, at least when the narrative begins. But as the man performing the accounting expands the temporal bounds of "it," the referential scope of the pronoun seems to enlarge itself as well.

Consider, for example, the following sentence; though "it" retains its sexual valence, it loses, through repetition, the stability of a specifiable referent:

You're with each other all day long and it keeps happening, the touches and smiles, and it adds up, it builds up, and you know where you'll be that night, you're talking and every now and then you think about it, no, you don't think, you just feel it as a kind of destination, what's coming up after you leave wherever you are all evening, and you're happy about it and you're planning it all, not in your head, really, somewhere inside your body, or all through your body, it's all mounting up and coming together so that when you get in bed you can't help it, it's a real performance, it all pours out. (127–28)

Dramatizing acts of cognition more than the episodes such acts try to organize, Davis's stories tend to center on scenes of interpersonal relation so deeply ensnared in their narrators' relentless efforts to scan, interpret, and evaluate that the partner in the encounter can seem blocked out, set aside, or made nominal by the overpresence of narratorial consciousness. As the sentence above aptly demonstrates, though, when that consciousness tries to assert the reality of something beyond itself, that something is frequently less an encounter with an actual other person than the somatic registration of an affect by which such encounters are experienced. Like a mode of thought in excess of the consciousness trying to describe it, such affect often qualifies or negates the sovereignty of consciousness. In the course of that negation, evoked above by making, then erasing claims for the cognitive agency of the narrator, "it" undergoes changes as well: "you think about it, no, you don't think, you just feel it"; "you're planning it all, not in your head really, somewhere inside your body"; "you can't help it, . . . it all pours out." Without losing its sexual freighting, "it" becomes the locus of resistance to the consciousness that tries to comprehend "it." In the process "it," as the object of encounter, ceases to occupy a determinate position either inside or outside the narrator. "It" names instead the excess produced in attempting to "break it down."

So when you read the subject's own breaking down, his dissolution into what you movingly call "a man without an infrastructure," as answered by the woman's gift of the shirt, which, in your words, "returns him to his skeleton" and, by doing so, "makes living on possible," I take your point but don't fully share this view of his response. Once the woman puts the shirt in his arms, you suggest, he "immediately begins to smell for her on" it, displacing her onto the shirt itself, which becomes a transitional object. But the text is less emphatic (as opposed to "Brokeback Mountain," for example,where Annie Proulx makes explicit the burden of a shirt as a figural skin), saying only "the soft cloth was full of her smell" and leaving in question whether he sniffs the scent out or merely takes it in. The difference matters only to the extent that you put so much weight on the shirt itself, making it into the fetish object central to the story as such: "there would be no narrative retrospect without the shirt," you maintain. But for me the shirt is not the story's object, in either sense of that word, and my claim depends on inserting the part of the sentence your quotation elides.

> And she was almost wild then, she reached up to a hook by the door and took an old shirt, a green and blue shirt from the hook, and put it in my arms, for me to take away, the soft cloth was full of her smell, and then we stood there close together looking at a piece of paper she had in her hand and I didn't lose any of it, I was holding it tight, that last minute or two, because this was it, we'd come to the end of it, things always change, so this was really it, over. (132)

Though the emotional drama plays itself out as the woman, "almost wild" with grief, gives the man the gift of her shirt, what seems to me more compelling is the sentence's resistance to that drama. Though he registers the shirt as "full of her smell," the man doesn't linger on it. Instead the shirt is displaced by attention to another and, in this context, stranger and, paradoxically enough, less legible object: "a piece of paper" that somehow suddenly appears in the woman's hand.

We learn nothing about this paper or why, after giving the man her shirt when she is said to be "almost wild," the woman then stands with the man close beside her while they look at the paper together. But two things seem significant here. First, the story begins with a glimpse of what might be this same piece of paper as a narrator, who immediately disappears from the text, sets the scene for the unnamed man's narrative: "He's sitting there staring at a piece of paper in front of him. He's trying to break it down" (127).

Nothing requires that this paper coincide with the "piece of paper" at the end, but in each case the paper seems extraneous, a detail in excess of narrative demand, and so indexical of the excess introduced by the labor of narrative accounting. Second, the first use of "it" in the story (in a phrase that inserts the title into the text) may take this "piece of paper" as its grammatical antecedent (and so may refer, metonymically, to what—if anything—is written on it): "He's sitting there staring at a piece of paper in front of him. He's trying to break it down." The "piece of paper" that appears at the story's end similarly calls forth a torrent of "its" while trying to affirm "it"s stability by insisting that "this was it . . . this was really it": "we stood there close together looking at a piece of paper she had in her hand and I didn't lose any of it, I was holding it tight, that last minute or two, because this was it, we'd come to the end of it, things always change, so this was really it, over." Is the "it" that the man holds tight here the shirt, the piece of paper, his experience with the woman, or the very fantasy of there being something, some "it," some object, for him to hold on to? The more emphatically he asserts that "this was it, . . . this was really it," the more difficult it becomes to believe that "it" could ever come into focus or attain the solidity he desires.

To that extent I agree with your claim that the story depicts an attempt to bring a "skeleton into being," but that skeleton, that framework for living on, is provided, in my view, less by the shirt as a transitional object allowing the man to live with affective mess than by the endless mutations of an "it" that takes on and casts off each particular referent that we or the man in the story would give it. In that sense "it"s negativity, "it"s resistance to fixed definition, sustains us. It keeps us coming back to the "piece of paper," to the narratives whereby we would square our accounts and make everything add up, but in which we encounter the persistent pressure of an unaccountable excess that breaks out from—and, in the process, breaks down—our efforts to break "it" down.

LB: I learned a lot from what you lay out here; I hadn't thought at all about the "it" or the papers. In any case, even if you would claim that all "againsts" are also "withs," the shirt is the second narrator's *objectum sexualis*, not mine: the story terminates with the sentence,

"So, I'm just thinking about it, how you can go in with $600, more like $1000, and how you can come out with an old shirt" (133). But I am loath to set up a competition among fetishes. This is partly because, in my view, not all invested-in objects are fetishes. It is possible to have a focalizing object that does not induce disavowal or whose structural function is not to enable it. Not all objects are equally overwhelming or overwhelming in the same way—but of course I would say this, as my claim throughout has been that an object is not one but a scene or fantasy setting that is living, moving, and available for multiple kinds of encounter. Your own reading of the "it" changes "it" across usages. Without revealing the "it" merely as structure, it emerges as a volatile agent that undergoes transformation in different contexts, with different implications. One might make the same observation about Freud's (1920/1955, 14–17) concept "fort/da": although the child's play with a top that he loses and repossesses repeatedly is widely read as a scene of play as mastery over loss, why not read it as a scene defined by a play with multiple consequences and risks—for example, the risks of possessing, ambivalence, being in control, being out of control, being alienated or dissociated, and/or the pleasures of cycling through these (see Lacan 1975/1988, 239)? Why not read the child's play as an experiment in potential form that does not seek out *a* form? Is it not possible that recontextualizing a problem shifts its conditions of extension even if *one* of its persistent conditions is its negativity? How to articulate structure and noise? What follows seeks to clarify these questions.

In classic psychoanalysis, a fetish has the double function of not representing negativity (by being a consoling distraction from the encounter with lack) and of representing it (by proliferating representations that stand for it). It offers and withholds cognitive control: the practice of acknowledgment plus disavowal phrased as "I know, but . . ." (Come to think of it, this is what you've been insisting about my position all along!) Had I been thinking in that idiom— I had chosen the passage about the shirt to initiate a discussion of nonsovereignty—the point would have been that the shirt is a failed fetish, that it cannot bear the organizing function to which it also aspires; despite the fact that the narrator's constant revisions, even in the very last instance, admit both his compulsion to come to an accounting and, more strongly, the futility of so doing. Disavowal would be a relief, but the mood is something else, anxious both for the event to amount to something and for the relief of a state of depletion. This is all technical, formal description; there is much we do not know about the affect.

All of the math in the world can't reendow the object with the encounter's clarifying wish. The narrator is overwhelmed that what remains is disorganization, that he cannot maintain the shirt even as a melancholic object, as a vehicle for sustaining the affective event beyond the live presence of the couple's dynamic. It should be no surprise, really, that the flatness of the story's end is the revelation of the shirt's existence beyond its capacity to sustain investment. So much of this story tracks the second narrator's persistent experience of forgetting the incident *while it is ongoing*. But to be with forgetting is not necessarily to be with the becoming-absent of something, just as, in chapter 2, I argued that loneliness is not a state of being alone; to forget is here to witness the conditioning of the object or scene itself, the psychic material's incomplete suppression, amid what I called the "dispersed environment of causes and pulses" that *can* get resolved in the fetish or symptom, but which here are not (Phillips 1994, 22–33).

The second narrator is both structured and destructured by the activity of such causes and pulses, experiencing the ways even a casually invested object can induce limerence, a flooding of unwonted ideation in the scene of attachment. There's a reason that an early state of erotic attachment is called in English "a crush": it crushes confidence, stability, intention. Intense attachment induces a nonsovereignty that confuses the habits of the pleasure, pain, and fantasy circuits. Both of these lovers are limerent, as far as we can tell, more blurting and playing than thinking and plotting, occupied by signs and phrases that are a little sourly unclear or not quite right — even at the end, when the woman is "wild," we don't *know* if it's with grief and/or desire and/or the release of the energy that a new formlessness engenders when an attachment shifts its genre. All we know is that they are trading in, and partly enjoying, and suffering, disorientation.

Compilations of thought like this are evidence for why, as Renata Salecl (2004) has argued, sexuality appears as style and why D. A.

Miller (2005) offers the concept of the *stylothete*, the subject for whom the achievement of style is as close as one gets to a genuinely sexually unanxious personhood. One's sexual style mobilizes the pleasure and the fear of nonsovereignty without dissipating, being out of control, or resolving it into a satisfying form. Sexual style involves practices that entrain, that pull oneself along, flung across rhythm and form. If it seeks solution, the resolution in form also involves solution's other sense, the loosening of the bonds of matter.

We know this second narrator as a set of styles. We know his styles through his failure to achieve style in relation—even in his narrative nonrelation with the first narrator, to whom he monologues. In "Break It Down" the sexual event produces in the second narrator countless encounters with a breakdown of style's capacity to float him—in sex, in dreams, while enacting norms, or in anxiety's performance of an out-of-controlness against which there can be no successful defense. Failed style produces multiple experiences of bodily weakness too (128, 131, 132). You focus on the narrator's attempts at control; I focus not only on the ways that he is always losing his grip but also on the ways he enjoys losing and having it, can't bear losing or having it, and is interested enough in it to induce a different form for encountering it. Breaking it down with the quiet narrator is another attempt to have a style with which he can live, and that desire may be all he, or anyone, brings to the table.

One thing that's crushed here, therefore, in the crush he has on his lover, is his capacity to disavow. And, I am claiming, this is identical to sensing his failure to achieve style. In being without an anchoring way of being, in being the subject of a slapstick sexuality absorbing the painful, the enjoyable, and the awkward, he faces so many perturbing things: the enigma of the lover; the impossibility of intersubjectivity; the inutility of sex as a building block for a knowing intimacy or a life; his aversion to knowing and being known; his fear of disaster and rejection; his sense of smallness, belatedness, contingency, and cognitive weakness. Knowing that thinking thinks him, he flails to keep up and fails to keep up. Belated to himself, he can't keep up with her either, in the most ordinary conversation, staged by Davis as that which must whiplash the reader's attention as well: "And she smiled at me and didn't stop talking and singing, something I said, she would sail into it, a snatch, for me, she would be gone from me a little ways, but smiling too, and tell me jokes, and I loved it but didn't exactly know what to do about it and just smiled back at her and felt slow next to her, just not quick enough" (127). She cannot keep up with herself either, in a sense: when she asks him, "Do I seem fat to you?" (130), she is delegating to him so many crises of self-encounter that he has no choice but to try to be game, to hold her together. He tries to stay in synch and to meet her worry, but they fail to repair whatever it was that produced her expression of a need to be held just so in the other's image. Yet it's her "fire," not her image, that gives him life. He senses that being entered by her energy means to "go on living," not in terms of immortality or ideality but in the live counterpoints and displacements of intimate relational time (130).

I concede that this gap between the fantasy of a structuring fetish and its failure to be both/and can be part of fetishism and can produce fake interrupts, as Freud explains, by producing objects available for devaluation and therefore fueling ongoing dramas of substitution. But being in the room with the chaos of styles that one brings to relationality and that relationality induces can also induce us to think differently about how we stay around our objects. Once the fetish is acknowledged as only one of many styles of relation, it is possible to imagine processes other than the rule of disavowal that do not merely invert it (elevating structure over mess or the opposite). "Break It Down" points to some ways to reoccupy the relation of structure to noise within rhythms of exchange. Once one acknowledges that one has not lost one's grip but never had it firmly or could have it, ever, in love or any structuring relation, then metaphors of holding and hoarding can be affectively reinvested, reconsidered, displaced, distributed, and diluted—and there is no choice, in the sense that one's forms are always being put next to other forms, other platforms for fantasy. Inducing transformative proximities like this is the task of politics and theory, as well as love. In so doing we are shifting our way of occupying negativity's hold on us.

LE: What you've written is tremendously helpful to me insofar as it raises two large questions central to our conversation: Does acknowledging a psychic or ideological fantasy necessarily change its hold on us? Might your faith in the power of acknowledgment (whether viewed as a cognitive or a discursive function) reproduce the fetishization it proposes to displace? I'd like to approach these questions by way of the sentences with which you end: "Once one acknowledges that one has not lost one's grip but never had it firmly or could have it, ever, in love or any structuring relation, then metaphors of holding and hoarding can be affectively reinvested, reconsidered, displaced, distributed, and diluted by being put next to other platforms for fantasy. This is the task of politics and theory, as well as love. In so doing we are shifting our way of occupying negativity's hold on us." I take your claim to be a strong one: not just that this act of "acknowledgment," like anything else that alters our relation to the world, will induce affective change as well but also, and more important, that acknowledging nonsovereignty, giving up the illusion of mastery or control, signally transforms our affective encounter with "ontological disorganization" and the "unruliness of the world." The promise of this narrative trajectory (acknowledgment recalibrates the hold on our affects of the metaphors of holding and hoarding; it allows us to let something go) grants cognition a truly striking degree of power over affect. But is affect really subordinate to acts of consciousness in this way? Are metaphors, especially those whose facilitations or pathways are largely unconscious, so readily dislodged?

To be sure, you say only that acknowledgment "can" allow for affective transformation, not that it will or must. But "acknowledgment" remains a master term in your account of the subject's potential for "shifting, remediating, and revisceralizing . . . threat." It holds the potential for something other than accustomed forms of affective response by making possible an escape from disavowal as a mode of defense against reality. Consider the following sentences that you've written in the preceding sections: "It matters that and how we acknowledge our affective discomposure in relation and the forms of misrecognition we improvise in ongoing negotiation with the sense of it"; "Once the fetish is acknowledged as only one of many styles of relation, it is possible to imagine principles other than the rule of disavowal that do not merely invert it." In each case (re)cognition makes possible shifts in affective experience by "induc[ing] us to think differently." But acknowledgment, as you yourself acknowledge, is essential to fetishism too, which, as you write, is "the practice of acknowledgment plus disavowal phrased as 'I know, but . . .'" As you rightly suggested, my concern is that your affirmation of the transformative potential inherent in acknowledgment may indeed keep company with a distinctive version of such fetishistic disavowal: the disavowal, precisely, of the limits of knowledge, and the limits of acknowledgment, in freeing us from "the rule of disavowal" with regard to our constitutive nonsovereignty.

It's not, of course, that you don't repeatedly acknowledge those very limits; but your acknowledgment is accompanied, if only implicitly, by a certain "but nonetheless." I'd venture to formulate it as follows: I know that the subject must live the incoherence that its constitutive nonsovereignty occasions, but nonetheless the conscious acknowledgment of our inevitable incoherence makes possible the affective transformation of our relations to the world. But insofar as affect exceeds our conscious regulation, mightn't that second clause disavow what's recognized by the first? Proposing the acknowledgment of nonsovereignty as a path toward affect's redistribution seems, in this context, to fetishize the knowledge whose limits you simultaneously maintain. And this is where we broach the problem for any politics that starts, as ours does, with the nonsovereignty of consciousness.

To see just what I mean by this, let's go back to the beginning of your response. You begin by maintaining, in a formulation with which I could hardly disagree (and whose deadpan humor made me laugh), "In any case, the shirt is the second narrator's *objectum sexualis*, not mine." I've known you long enough to affirm unconditionally that this is true. But, of course, I never suggested that we interpret the shirt as *your* sexual object, only that your reading had the effect of "turning [the shirt] into the fetish object central to the story as such" and that it did so in a way that the story, at least in my view, doesn't sustain. Your account of the shirt, your reckoning of its value to the man and the story both, transforms it into a fetish *for them*, makes it, as you say, the second narrator's *objectum sexualis*. This is the claim from which I demur; I don't see the shirt as his fetish or as the fetish of the story itself (though in the context of fetishism,

I love the fact that you describe it as a skin that returns him to his skeleton, filling his empty space with bone). While "Break It Down" concludes, as you note, with a sentence that returns to the shirt — "So, I'm just thinking about it, how you can go in with $600, more like $1000, and how you can come out with an old shirt" (133) — it's impossible to know from this sentence and its indeterminate tone ("So, I'm just thinking about it . . .") whether the "old shirt" is an object of the narrator's over- or underinvestment, whether it indicates, as you write, that "the narrator is overwhelmed that he cannot maintain the shirt even as a melancholic object," or whether it is merely one figure among others, as contingent to him as it is to the woman at the moment when she puts it in his arms, for everything he judges incapable of representing "it."

In this latter view, toward which I'm inclined, his persistence in attempting to break "it" down, to offer an adequate accounting, does not, as I see it, necessarily "admit . . . the futility of so doing." For the man, to the very end, will substitute measuring, mental calculation ("I'm just thinking about it"), and the production of theory (a theory of value) for the absence of a final *measure* of value, for the lack, that is, of an apprehensible "it" susceptible to the cognitive measure some god of mathematics could guarantee. That god of mathematics is nothing less than God as the final accountant, the Other who balances the books, and so the hypostatized ground for a faith in measurement as a value itself, in thought as equal to the task of reckoning, as capable of "breaking it down." But how can we take the measure of thought as the measure with which we reckon when the primal attachments that form and deform it escape our every reckoning?

"We enter a realm of crude fetishism," writes Nietzsche, "when we summon before consciousness the basic presuppositions of the metaphysics of language — in plain talk, the presuppositions of reason. Everywhere reason sees a doer and doing; it believes in will as *the* cause; it believes in the ego, in the ego as being, in the ego as substance, and it projects this faith in the ego-substance upon all things — only thereby does it first *create* the concept of 'thing'" (1954/1976, 482–483). If the fetish here produces the concept of the thing as a corollary to reason's assertion of a substance or agent responsible for willing, then it makes good sense that Nietzsche, shortly after this passage, should write, "I am afraid we are not rid of God because we still have faith in grammar" (483). God alone is the guarantee of reason as linguistic organization, even if God, like the subject, is merely the literalization of grammatical "voice" (de Man 1979, 18). Isn't this related to what Lacan maintains when he notes that Descartes had to turn to God to secure the field of knowledge? "What Descartes means, and says," Lacan insists, "is that if two and two make four it is, quite simply, because God wishes it so" (1973/1978, 225). Our faith in thought's ability, by *acknowledging* nonsovereignty, to account for it in such a way that it enters into the count we produce of ourselves and our relations, thereby inducing a transformation that rescripts us at the level of affect, may bespeak a similar fetishistic belief in the power of knowledge to operate on what knowledge doesn't govern in the first place. To that extent, it may disavow the insistence of the unconscious and the Real.

You write, "It is possible to have a focalizing object that does not induce disavowal or whose structural function is not to enable it." As an example, you cite my own attention to the metamorphoses of "it": "Your own reading of the 'it' changes 'it' across usages," you assert. "Without revealing the 'it' merely as structure, 'it' emerges as a volatile agent that itself undergoes transformation in different contexts." But my point, in fact, is that "it" as the second narrator's "focalizing object" *does* reveal a structure. Figuring his reification of the unattainable *objet a*, "it" is the structural counterpart to the narrator's faith in thought. In this sense the multiplications of "it" disavow its nonexistence as a comprehensive totality. Isn't that, however, the function of any "focalizing object"? By organizing reality, by creating the sense of logical relation, it disavows the absence of an a priori ground that might uphold such organization: the absence, to return to your metaphor, of a "skeleton" supporting reality itself. The "focalizing object" *produces* the "skeleton" that, in your words, "makes living on possible." But that living on requires the continuous disavowal of the Real. The Real can be readily acknowledged, of course; we can "know" that the skeleton, the framework, sustaining reality won't stand up. Nonetheless, we continue to believe in the framework that permits us to dismantle that framework itself as no more than the product of fantasy.

Here, in my view, our readings of the text converge with the second narrator's attempts to theorize and determine "it"s value. That is, we go into the story hoping to articulate the consequences of non-sovereignty and come out perhaps with our own conceptual equivalents of "an old shirt," which is to say, with thoughts that affirm the efficacy of thought, the power of knowledge or acknowledgment to change what exceeds its scope. This does not amount (to stay with the mathematical metaphor a bit) to a corrigible error in thinking about either nonsovereignty or Davis's text; instead it measures (that concept again) a limit intrinsic to thought. For the second narrator in "Break It Down," accounting is the fetish intended to organize the disorganization of "it"—a disorganization that follows from his initial association of "it" with a sexual encounter that deroutinizes his life. (Should we note that the idiom, "break it down," refers not only to the explanatory function evinced by logical parsing but also, in rap, to dancing and, not surprisingly, to sexual acts?) Though he theorizes "it"s instability, "it"s ceaseless recomputations of value, his theorization takes for granted that theory or thought is adequate to "it"s measure. In this sense *theory* becomes the skeleton, the fetishized bone that would fill up his emptiness and enable his living on.

Though not every object of psychic investment constitutes a fetish, those that sustain a fantasy on which "living on" depends, those that operate by denying lack while expressing, through negation, its threat, *do* function fetishistically and deserve to be read as such. I proposed earlier that "politics [is] the fantasy, when you break it down, of breaking down figures of fantasy." In this we can see where politics and theory might usefully coincide: in their shared resistance to reification, their common identity as negative practices that dismantle the fantasy of identity. Despite my doubts about acknowledgment as a path to affective change, I do invest in the fantasy, both personally and pedagogically, of breaking fantasy down. Not because I believe that a life without fantasy is possible or desirable (how could it be desirable, after all, except by way of fantasy?) but rather because the reification of fantasy as reality, as what de Lauretis calls the "literality, or referentiality, [that] is a mainstay of political discourse" (de Lauretis 2011, 257), does violence both to those who reify themselves through attachment to it and to those made to figure the insistence of the Real that would rupture it from within. That rupture, for me, corresponds to the drive's repetitive intrusion on fantasy but also to the imperative of politics as negativity, as dissent from the world as given. As opposed to the political imaginary, with its fantasy (an indispensable fantasy) of constituting community, it expresses the Real of politics as the breaking from and of what is. And in that I find "the task of politics and theory, as well as love."

LB: One of your styles of response, Lee, is to pose some version of the question "Is *x* necessarily so?" Then, if you can show that *x* is not necessarily so, you return to your structuring view, for to you, a structure is necessarily so. You write, though, "I do invest in the fantasy, both personally and pedagogically, of breaking fantasy down." From one perspective, this is something like what the second narrator might say, which I know wouldn't bother you, since your tendency is to argue that we cannot not want the control and repair over relation that we also cannot achieve. But it also opens onto what I am claiming, which is that if the multiplication of orientations toward negativity cannot enable the antinomies of life to appear as consistencies, it can change the consequences of negativity's work and therefore the object or scene of encounter itself. Does this mean that you *do* invest in the fantasy that a breakdown of fantasy might point to a nonrepetitive libidinal or political outcome, a transformation in what structure does, by virtue of how it appears? Or is it that you fantasize breaking fantasy, in its binding to representation? Or . . . ? I am trying to understand how you understand the implications of your investment.

To me, and to us mutually, I think, some things *are* necessarily so: that the subject is the scene of encounter of the productive or negating disciplines of the world *and* of the ordinary work of taking up a position in form that is never fully complete, never consistent, always elliptical, noisy, and threateningly incoherent. At the same time, we agree that gestures that interrupt the patterns through which one predictably makes one's way in life do not "readily dislodge" anything or change a structure tout court, making or destroying a world. But that just looks like the old structure-agency impasse. It also does not mean that one's affective patterns represent coherently the totality of one's actions or the totality of structure. Shifts in the atmospheres through which fantasy finds anchors in symbolization, shifts that I associate with political struggles over imaginaries and the reproduction of life, may not transform what a structure is—since fantasy is itself a structure within the negative—but they shift what fantasy does, how it arcs, what it reaches, and what's available to be in play. The subject is an effect of such play. This is why scenes of love and loss, scenes of an overwhelmed sensorium pushed to improvise action (flailing about making and unmaking worlds), are key to assessing how we do and can live with negativity. Why is love, the encounter with relationality, *not* always traumatic, while always overwhelming? To get at this question requires elaborating a different sense of negativity's relation to relation.

I've been phrasing this as whether and how it matters what we do. If one's capacity to disavow is crushed, if the fetish fails at maintaining its own processes, one can always wait for the next train (of ideation) and begin again, taking up form with amnesiac hope. Or one can welcome the next breakdown of fantasy as a confirming reencounter with one's disappointment with the world and/or oneself. But one can also discover that one has already made different kinds of room to move and shifted potentials for moving along with the unbearable. Affect affects worlds and is impacted by them; the disjunction between affect, the event of its worlding (when it seeks a world), and anything like consciousness makes possible different encounters with oneself and one's objects. Moving differently with affect is therefore not the same as pretending that a drama of decision changes things permanently or fundamentally. It involves discovering and inhabiting disturbances in the relation between one's affects and one's imaginaries for action. That discovery is the site of potentially recontextualizing creativity.

But, as I have argued previously, it is not as though structuration comes from inside, and it is my attention to multiple kinds of exterior force, I think, that induces your staging of me as more bound to the signifier than you are and to the sensual, historical experience of encounter. I think that's correct too, insofar as I don't perceive that to call the world's modes of negation and antagonism "structural" makes them structural in the same way, or an expression of the drives, as you have attested. In chapter 2, through Sedgwick and Cavell, I suggested that acknowledgment, what we do in the sustained presence of an object, can extend a nonmastering relation to the enigma of that object that performs our obligation to it by way of a looseness that, from the perspective of drama, can constitute a formally comic scene or make routes within the impossible. I appreciate that, to you, this wedge can seem like a hedge against confronting the drama of negativity within the setting fantasy provides for enlisting the attachment to attachment. But the drama of negativity takes on many valences. As fantasy provides settings for enduring relationality, different objects and scenes produce different potentials for living with negativity.

Here's another walk around the situation. Christopher Bollas (1987: 4) defines the "unthought known" as "the reliving through language of that which is known but not yet thought." It exerts a pressure that the subject senses as an ongoing intuiting of one's own and the world's own rhythms and pulses; it is not the same kind of knowing that carries with it a sense of mastered truth. This means that those norms delivered to us as truths, for example, are not just copied in us as truths but as the aspirations of power in an atmosphere of potential action where it might have been otherwise. The unthought known is an anchoring pressure of a relation to an object world and, within relationality, an insistent proposition about it with whose patternings the subject identifies as an orientation loosely moored to the explicit event. One might even call it a structure. It may be related to Laplanche's "enigmatic signifier" too, the unstated erotic pleasure that places us in relation not only to what we have been casting as the subject's unbearable access to his own radical unrepresentability but also to the sensual pleasures of relationality itself (Laplanche 1992, 160).

So far we have been pointing to the subject's unbearable encounter with her radical incoherence, her trembling out-of-synchness with her fantasy of herself in the world, and the fantasies of sovereignty that seek to shift—you would say "master"—the dramatic nonrelation so that the encounter with it might not be absolutely defeating, repeating, and depleting. Folding pleasure into the structure of the unbearable would recast the shape of the thing that we have agreed to mean by *structure*. In this view the structure to which the subject returns is organized not only by a movement between negativity and disavowal but also by a negativity that is sensed, inarticulately, as a condition of being in the world a certain way, that is, as a feeling of displacement that is inevitable, nonsovereign, and at the same time a pressure to which the subject remains attached. It is pleasurable insofar as it induces desire to be in the neighborhood of the object; it is overwhelming insofar as it reveals the necessity of relationality itself. "The individual's first and forever-recurring loss, in Freud's view, is not of the object but of the fantasy of self-sufficiency, of being everything to oneself" (Phillips 1993, 99).

This is the kind of thing to which I have been pointing: to the sense of being primally unmastered by need that one senses but does not know, in your sense of knowledge as mastery; a sense clustered with the sense of a need for the objects or scenes that hold up the world and pleasure in that need (not happiness, but pleasure, the form of enduring repetition itself).

I believe you have predicted this move. When you call sex "the site where desire, for all its potential mobility, remains fixed to a primal attachment that alone makes our objects appear as desirable," do you not mean that sex forces you, primally, to want an object? That's what makes it a drive; pleasure and "wanting" here have nothing to do with liking, or idealizing, or any particular experience. Likewise I see sex as an arena where a cluster of excited inclinations to discover a (dis)place within attachment is played out. It is a place where the trembling of one's penetration by relationality is always revealed, even when no one else is in the room. It is a scene in which one enjoys the risk of moving through a field of ambivalence, resistance, and interest.

I keep thinking of the pathos of our second narrator's tone, his insistence on extending the always reconfiguring situation to a time in the penumbra of the live relation. "I guess you get to a point where you look at that pain as if it were there in front of you three feet away lying in a box, an open box, in a window somewhere," he says, acting as a witness at the funeral of love. The pain is "hard and cold," the second narrator says, "like a bar of metal. You just look at it there and say, All right, I'll take it, I'll buy it. That's what it is. Because you know all about it before you even go into this thing. You know the pain is part of the whole thing" (132–33). Renting space in the vast "shadow of the object," he stays there by multiplying objects, moving between a thing that can be seen through but would shatter if moved through and a thing that's solid, is all outside or inside. He is reexperiencing the primal abandonment after which the subject is launched into a life of crafting relationality with objects he moves with, moving in synch and syncope. The bar of metal is his mettle, his unspent hoard of potential and immanent relationality, and it has a crushing and animating weight. Desire's binding and unbinding circuits are not only *not* disavowed by his gestures, they are also acknowledged in the atmosphere around the question "Why doesn't that pain make you say, I won't do it again?" (133).

Is this a rhetorical question? We don't know. If his variations do not matter to him—if he is doing everything he can not to give up his "libidinal position"—he might be trying to disavow by mastering. He might be happy as a fetishist who enjoys the constraints he has embraced against the encroachments of disorder. He might incline to misrecognize closure as a form of openness, of sickly, necessary hope. He might also sense that no form, no answer to the question will solve the problem of living, will allow him to stay in the scene of desire to produce, at minimum, the comfort of self-encounter and of encounter with the world's potentiality for changing what the intractable can mean.

To me, regardless, such a refusal of form's adequacy is a central premise of antinormative politics, without which there is no refusal of the social negation that seeks to capture one's own negativity. Identity is the "it" broken down through the recognition that one's beloved objects, including oneself, are placeholders for an ever-evolving set of desires and forces; facing "it" induces the discomfort and excitement in being with all that and forces a reconsideration of what Spivak would call the foundational "lack of fit" not just within but with the world on which one nonetheless also converges and toward which one cannot, nonetheless, not incline (Spivak 1987, 207).

This suggests that one can sense the breakdown of form in this story as a different kind of event from what you project. Our second narrator is seeing as clearly as can be seen the political form of the question of pain. He pushes toward a change that is not more of the same and does not see that as an internal shift but one that must take place in rhythms of sustaining relational inclination, which is something different from a sovereign thought or a plan. We know this because he has turned to another in front of whom to recite his sums, his *summa*.

Why else, after all, is the story told to a silent listener? Perhaps he hopes that the listener will shut up and nod, so that he can pretend that his monologue is a genuine exchange. There is something flat in the story's staging of it too, as though the title captures the first narrator's last moments of attention before spacing out as the man spins out his process of being unmastered by what you call faith in cognition. Perhaps the nonencounter of the sexual encounter has moved from mouth to ear, as Foucault would have predicted, and he's once again monologuing, just this time externally, forcing his internal states onto someone who has consented to be there. But at the same time, in giving his story over, consciously or not, he opens the possibility of its crumbling in front of another—no longer in the trembling of sex but in the expansive uncuratedness of conversation, a scene inevitably of nonsovereign relationality as such.

Depletion is also necessary for unsticking to a fantasy that is no longer working. In addition to the bodily pleasures that you detail, the phrase *break it down* refers to what happens to a theatrical set after a dramatic performance; it also entails a request for a speaker to simplify something complicated. Not just a request: out of context, as a title, "Break It Down" is in the imperative, which, Barthes writes, is always the *mood* of the claim for love. "Break It Down," then, also amounts to a love letter to love, addressed not only to the need for a reparative object but also to the need for access to the mood of the broken fantasy. As it shatters, the story proliferates into arcs. Is this cluster of displacements close to what you meant by the fantasy of breaking fantasy down?

LE: You read the question I posed earlier ("Does acknowledging a psychic or ideological fantasy necessarily change its hold on us?") as manifesting what you see as a "style" of response that allows me—illegitimately?—to "return to [my] structuring view," by which I understand you to mean: allows me to affirm, in a given instance, the presence of a structural determination. "For to you," as you put it, "a structure is necessarily so." If I claim that I don't "return" to such a view, it's because I don't think I ever left it (which, given my position, should hardly come as much of a surprise). I do believe that what I call structures are "necessarily so"; it's precisely that belief that leads me to define them as structures in the first place. To the extent that my phrasing was misleading (perhaps a consequence of the irony implicit in the grammatical form of the rhetorical question), let me clarify it here. Acknowledging a psychic or ideological fantasy, the act you recurrently formulate as allowing the movement, the change in atmosphere, that you construe as potentially transformative, does not, in my view, release us from the hold of a structuring fantasy. This is why the question of the fetish seemed to impose itself on us earlier, for the fetish makes clear that acknowledging a fantasy does not dissolve its power. The structure of the fantasy doesn't coincide with the image (not even the image of *itself*) that the fantasy produces. If fantasy, in other words, always entails the production of an image, the image may be changed without affecting the structure (for Lacan, a *defensive* structure) within which it occurs. We can fantasize, as fetishism demonstrates, that we "know" our relation to fantasy, but the image of the fantasy we believe we "know" differs from that of the fantasy we enact in believing that we know it.

Thus the process of changing the fantasy image, of opening the potential for psychic mobility through the unblocking of desire, may itself reinforce a fantasy structure by occluding our fixation to *desire itself* as a defense against the drive (where the drive enacts the structure that desire, through the lure of its objects, conceals). Fantasy, as the Lacanian matheme suggests ($ <> a$), always relates to *objet a* as object/cause of desire (Lacan 1966/2006, 653). And this underscores the stakes involved in thinking about sex, negativity, and politics by cutting to the heart of the question of change in relation to the unconscious. Displacements of our objects in the metonymic sequence distinctive of desire do not bespeak changes in our structuring fantasy even if they induce a new "atmosphere" in which that fantasy plays itself out. And it's not as if we could somehow function—psychically, socially, or politically—in the absence of such a fantasy frame, as Slavoj Žižek points out in his reading of Lacan's "les non-dupes errent" (2000, 323). We rely for our reality as subjects on the fantasy image by which we flesh out and deny our constitutive division. That's why we find ourselves torn between the defensive stabilization our fantasies perform and the negativity of the drive that disrupts them, a drive that comes to consciousness only as a *fantasy* of negativity, reinforcing the ego once more. In neither politics nor sex do we engage the positivity of relation; both open instead onto the impossibility inherent in the *encounter*: the impossibility, that is, of confronting the other as positivized in the object without *also* confronting the unbearable negativity that the object can never sublate and that fantasy can never subsume.

That's why you rightly distance yourself from any reading of your investment in acknowledgment as faith in the subject's self-determination on the basis of rational analysis. "Moving differently with affect," you write, "is therefore not the same as pretending that a drama of decision changes things permanently or fundamentally." But your very next sentence produces, as I see it, a certain complication: "It [i.e., moving differently with affect] involves discovering and inhabiting disturbances in the relation between one's affects and one's imaginaries for action." To the extent, however, that affect and action are intimately related (affect naming at once the somatic manifestation of psychic activity and the subject's relation to bodily action), the concept of "moving" differently with affect raises the question of just what agency would generate such movement. Logically it can't be affect itself, but it isn't, as I think we both agree, the subject of cognition either. This makes the relation between "moving differently with affect" and the "drama of decision" uncertain. Is the change in one's way of moving with affect produced by a "drama of decision" or not—which is to say, is it the result of an acknowledgment on the part of the subject that is then supposed to have the ability to change its affective experience? If such movement springs from no "drama of decision" but arises instead from the "discovery" (by the conscious or the unconscious subject?) of "disturbances" (an affective discovery therefore) in the relation between affect and "one's imaginaries for action" (which is also to say, between affect and one's fantasy of sovereignty), then how is this movement (which is going to move us "differently" through affect) different from the innumerable micro-adjustments that regulate our response to the "atmosphere" (what Eve would call the "weather") in which we live our affective lives? Or is moving differently with affect achieved by a "drama of decision" after all, but a drama of decision that we recognize (or, to return to the key word, acknowledge) as necessarily provisional?

And how, in this context, should we interpret your invocation of Bollas's "unthought known"? Bollas uses this concept to refer to a property of the ego and, more precisely, to a property of the unconscious ego that includes the "inherited disposition," or what he also calls the "personality" that exists, according to his argument, *before* the infant's birth. The "unthought known" in his account is capable of being brought to consciousness. "A psychoanalysis will bring the 'unthought known' into thought," he writes. "Through psychoanalysis the ego is encountered and known" (Bollas 1987, 9). Indeed so strong is his commitment to bringing this unthought known to thought, so far does its reach extend, that the unthought known gets bound up for Bollas with "a recollection of the person's ontogenesis" and so with the baby's capacity to "express his knowing of his being through fantasy, thought and object relating" (60). In this regard it speaks to Bollas's filiations with Jung in the latter's "humanistic" resistance to the negativity of Freud. Andrew Samuels, for instance, describes that resistance in the following terms:

> Freud's view of human psychology is a bleak one and, given the history of the twentieth century, it seems reasonable. But Jung's early insistence that there is a creative, purposive, non-destructive core of the human psyche finds echoes and resonances in the work of psychoanalytic writers like Milner and Rycroft, and in Winnicott's work on play. . . . Jung's argument that the psyche has knowledge of what is good for it, a capacity to regulate itself, and even to heal itself, takes us to the heart of contemporary expositions of the "true self" such as that found in Bollas's recent work." (Samuels 1997, 5)

But such a view of the subject's "being" (or of fantasy itself as an expression of that being instead of as a mode of defense against the knowledge of its loss) attests to the insistence of a set of beliefs at odds with the version of psychoanalysis within which my own work proceeds.

And that's because I, like you, don't believe that "structuration comes from inside"—or not, at any rate, from "inside" some fixed disposition that precedes the subject's encounter with otherness. Rather it is the subject who "comes from" the encounter with those structures that leave their decisive inscription on its psychically potentialized soma. That, of course, explains why the "enigmatic signifier" matters so much for Laplanche—and even for Lacan, who used the term earlier. And it's why for you and me alike the unbearable encounter of the subject with its radical incoherence works *against* recuperations of "being." The fantasy of sovereignty succumbs not only to the recognition of non-self-sufficiency, as your quotation from Phillips indicates, but also to the necessity of the subject's emergence as the division, the bar of signification, that it repeatedly tries to rise above in the sexual (non)relation.

In this sense I completely agree when you characterize the subject as attached to the negativity that marks its "condition of being in the world." I'd call that attachment to negativity primal, for that negative condition becomes the ground for the subject's ability to signify itself. But that attachment doesn't, in my view, simply ground itself in "pleasure"; it carries instead the force of what's "beyond" the pleasure principle: a compulsion, a repetition, a drive that escapes the affirmation of the ego to which the experience of pleasure conforms (what you evoke as the "form of enduring repetition itself"). For the same reason I don't read the subject's attachment to negativity as generating "desire to be in the neighborhood of our objects." Negativity repeats the primal division that makes the subject "one" only to the extent that the subject imagines that it can refind itself in the signifier whose "unary stroke" divides it (Lacan 1973/1978, 218). The fantasmatic object, then, the object of desire, *positivizes* the subject's lack and thereby secures the subject precisely as subject of castration, as subject of desire. But the insistent attachment to negativity expresses the failure, the insufficiency, of every such positivization. And this insufficiency is structurally determined by the Symbolic order of language in which, by (re)finding our objects repeatedly, we perform, through that very repetition, our refusal of the object as adequate to filling the gap, the division that we are. It's not that we renounce our objects, abandon the Symbolic, and plunge into lack, but rather that our objects express the entanglement of attachment and negativity. This is where you and I come together in thinking about sex "as an arena where a cluster of excited inclinations to discover a (dis)place within attachment is played out."

But what can we do with this negativity that won't disavow what it does to us? We both agree that refusing to accept the adequacy of given forms, which is also to say, the sufficiency of any social positivization, grounds antinormative politics. Insofar as that politics resists the fantasmatic coherence to which those forms lay claim, it always works to break down the fantasy of the object that, to borrow your phrase, "will solve the problem of living." Just here, however, the fantasy of breaking down fantasy returns. For every investment in negativity as a potentializing instrument—as the means of breaking down fantasy (and, with it, the *structural* immobility concealed by the movement of its *images* or *scenes*)—fetishistically disavows its own fantasy structure, which commits it to another version of "solv[ing] the problem of living." Such an investment remains, like theory itself, a defense against the breaking down it simultaneously desires—a defense precisely to the extent that it remains embedded in desire and therefore in the fantasmatic displacement of the drive. Isn't this related to what de Man (1986) had in mind with his notion of the "resistance to theory": that negativity, however persistent, doesn't persist when we try to harness it to a known or predictable form—or doesn't, at any rate, persist in the form we expect it to take in that harness?

For just this reason your focus on the performative context of the second narrator's musings strikes me as crucially important. It opens a set of questions at the very core of our conversation by broaching the issue of the join between conversation and relationality. Once again the textual object with which we anchor our dialogue has captured us unexpectedly in its frame. Is the object (for us, for the second narrator, or even for the first) encountered as something outside ourselves, or does it insist on the fantasy of "relation" as a way of resisting encounter as such? Though I don't think conversation is "inevitably" a "scene . . . of nonsovereign relationality" (all too often—perhaps even in Davis's text—it becomes the fantasmatic scene of sovereign assertion), I do think it marks the site of a potential encounter with the unbearable, with the otherness that permits no relation despite our best efforts to construct one.

That threat of the unbearable lurks in the figure of pain as a bar of metal. I'd like us to linger on that bar for a while, because I see it as evoking the irreducible otherness that makes relation as such impossible. It speaks to the element in encounter that we try to bend to relational value, try to subsume to the economy of relation, when it marks, in fact, the impenetrability of what eludes our measure: "You can't measure it, because the pain comes after and it lasts longer" (133). If the second narrator maintains nonetheless that the pain "doesn't . . . make you say, I won't do it again" (133), that reflects his desire to conceive the pain—however obdurate or hard it may be—as an object with which, through repeated encounter, he can enter into relation by turning it into an object of knowledge (which all his objects become): "Because you know all about it before you even go into this thing. You know the pain is part of the whole thing" (133). As the bar to relation that has to submit to the bartering of relationality ("You just look at it there and say, All right, I'll take it, I'll buy it" [133]), the bar of metal, "lying in a box, an open box, in a window somewhere" (132–33), serves as a window onto the encounter with relation's negativity.

LB: Conversation does require nonsovereignty, whether or not it feels otherwise or is marked manifestly by controlling gestures. This is why, beneath the skin, a defensive sense so often accompanies one's inclination to susceptibility, and why any encounter's aspiration to synchrony is haunted by the threat of foreclosure games, even one's own, whose styles might manifest in patter that dominates, cares, or inattends. But as any genre brings with it metal bars, or dramas of desire, risk, and potential failure, the attachment to attaching is also an investment in other things that incite not control but a kind of cruising, a seeking to see what happens in relation without caring much to know what *precisely* the object is or who one is in relation to it. Contradictory aims are both resolved in the management of negativity and remain unsolved too, as they constitute the very density of a situation's hologram. (Your reading of Bollas walks by this claim about the systematic pressure of the affective nonknowledge that moves us within attachment; it's a place where we'll have to diverge.)

Another way to say this is that, if to you the "fantasmatic object . . . the object of desire, *positivizes* the subject's lack," to me, that object is also not an object but a scene, a setting for actions, a discontinuous space that appears navigable for moving around awkwardly, ambivalently, and incoherently, while making heuristic sense of what's becoming-event. This setting is what Laplanche calls "fantasy." So, because I see the structure of the object as less tight or homogeneous than your staging of it suggests, I don't think that "otherness . . . permits no relation despite our best efforts to construct one." I think it permits no neutral, stable, or consistent relation, but some relation-in-movement, more affective and sensed in the penumbra of the manifest content of the contact invested with images. If the encounter can never fully be governed by the "potentializing instrument" of a reparative genre, whether from sex, politics, or theory, the open question for me, then, much more than for you, is about how relationality gestures beyond itself toward altered settings for the hits and misses. The experimentality in worlding complicates the space of the encounter with negativity; it's where I locate political potentiality.

I'm playing this out polemically partly to increase the noise level within the psychoanalytic idiom of debate into which we've gotten ourselves. At times I think we risk losing the big picture, which to me does not involve a fantasy of making a big picture of a repaired world of happy lovers, adequate storytellers, and properly recognized beings. It involves, as theorists, taking on the overdetermination of encounter in the staging of reparative fantasy—which points to something in addition to allegory. This returns us to the question of narrative.

As you've pointed out, my ongoing interest is in at once attending to the story of the postsovereign and the nonsovereign—the state of the collective world of distributed power, values, norms, affects, and practices and the states of affect that traverse singular and collectively emergent sensoriums. Thinking about "structure" less as the insistence of the Real and more as that which organizes diverse and contradictory systemic forces, I've been arguing that the nonidentity of nonrelation in these different registers allows scenic shifts in addition to the theater of minor adjustments to which you refer. Negativity might not change, but the worlding of it does.

But this optimism does not entail binding the negative to better objects. In a different version of this essay I might have started by noting that Davis's récit takes place after a vacation, a vacation from work. From what I hear, vacations are also experiments in nonsovereignty, attempts to enjoy unproductivity, dehabituation, and fantasy by disturbing one's usual dynamics, objects and scenes, and affective registers. (I am laughing at this description, which refuses to take a vacation from abstraction.)

Nonetheless the intense presence of the capitalist imaginary in Davis's récit points to the impossibility of vacating the structuring fantasy: one can leave work but not the dreamwork. Our second narrator's fantasy remains saturated with the language of property and of data, of the individual and the dividual. Not only that, but the productive ordinary reappears in the monologue's pathetic echo of the optimism for nonsovereign sexuality that has legitimated sexual hookups without property relations since the heyday of progressive heterosexual practice after '68, when the hope was that the mutual reorganization of intimacy and productivity would induce new forms of life. A new form of life would restructure the work of structure. The desire for this released a lot of reparative creativity in the 1960s. Some of it endures and develops; most of it didn't. "Break It Down" is a eulogy to how accidentally bad the sexual revolution's math could be. But accidents are information: just as a vacation involves openness to accident, so to talk about love, as Barthes wrote, is always to talk about the centrality of accident to love's very structure.

But if "Break It Down" rehearses the inability to produce an emancipatory labor theory of affective value, the straight-dominated world's release into a mode of sexual life without guarantees no longer allows the easy narrative foreclosure that would disavow intimacy's induction of pleasure, torture, confusion, and boredom, especially when, as in this case, lovers peel away from teleology-flavored plots, discarding romantic resolution without discarding their need for encounter. The question is, then, how to induce another story, or world, for the dynamic in which the negating and ecstatic burst of the subject that Nancy (2003) calls "shattered love" negotiates its patterns and accidents. Again this other story is not what *appears* in "Break It Down," but the flat ending points to it, pressing us to imagine elliptically, beyond the second narrator's broken rhythm and his restless imaging. Note in the following passage, by the way, the story's prophetic staging of our very impasse:

And finally the pictures go and these dry little questions just sit there without any answers and you're left with this large heavy pain in you that you try to numb by reading, or you try to ease it by getting out into public places where there will be people around you, but no matter how good you are at pushing that pain away, just when you think you're going to be all right for a while, that you're safe, you're kind of holding it off with all your strength and you're staying in some little bare numb spot of ground, then suddenly it will all come back, you'll hear a noise, maybe it's a cat crying or a baby, or something else like her cry, you hear it and make that connection in a part of you you have no control over and the pain comes back so hard that you're afraid, afraid of how you're falling back into it again and you wonder, no, you're terrified to ask how you're ever going to climb out of it. (130–31)

Two things interest me here. One is fear of the question. The second is the presence of the phatic, of noise.

Our narrator is not terrified of being alone, exactly. He is terrified of being left with a question that he can also not bear to pose, a question so overwhelming that it fails to become genuinely interrogative.

For some reason, by which I mean, in response to the pressure of inarticulate affect, this makes me want to close by gesturing toward mourning. In "Break It Down," mourning is a scene of being left with a question in the form of a flattened-out statement, a question about the fading of the object of desire and its dissolution into noise, a feral cry. When Davis writes about love, the scene of the actual ongoing encounter is boring, overwhelming, too tender for words, inefficient, delayed, gestural, aspirational, and habitable only through repetitions that allow the viscera to settle, for moments, in the space their repetitions make. The genre of the elliptical question allows what's dead, live, and excessive in love to occupy the same space, to be in the same story, which is the same thing as in the same scene or situation. In "How Shall I Mourn Them?" she imagines beloveds in terms of the gestures that made them characters to her, expressed in images of a characteristic movement:

Shall I keep a tidy house, like L.?
Shall I develop an unsanitary habit, like K.?

Shall I sway from side to side a little as I walk, like C.?
Shall I write letters to the editor, like R.?
Shall I retire to my room often during the day, like R.?
Shall I live alone in a large house, like B.?
Shall I treat my husband coldly, like K.?
Shall I give piano lessons, like M.?
Shall I leave the butter out all day to soften, like C.?
Shall I have problems with typewriter ribbons, like K.?
  (Davis 2010, 697)

Here attachment is encrypted in a question that is not quite a riddle and not quite rhetorical. The sentences end twice, with a period and question mark that abbreviate and extend the encounter with the scene of encounter with the object. The object of attachment isn't standing still for a portrait, either, but emerges in movement, like the cat, baby, lover, placeholders all, encountered as a direct and yet mediated impact. The sound they emit is also not a question, a demand, or an expressive autobiography but a repetitive noise that raises the specter of a singular relationality. Davis captures here not the love found in conventional narrative but something else that's open, to be encountered queasily and interestedly.

Davis also emblematizes this alternative orientation toward narrative in "The Center of the Story," where, "unlike a hurricane, this story has no center" (173). In "The Center of the Story," a narrator appears as a consciousness that cruises potential sites of interest that can never fully anchor all of the tale's elements and intensities. Here Davis finds an alternative to the narrative norm structured by the drama of making and undoing—breaking down—a complication. Everything moves, as there is no center structuring life as an unbroken event. This helps me see why Davis opens up not the futurity of the will-have-been that you associate with narrative, but the sense that to call something narrative *rather* than scenic is itself to enact a fantasy that there is something beyond the ongoing, with all of the anachronistic force it bears. This returns us to our discussion in chapter 1 of whether narrative requires expectations of temporal extension and satisfaction.

Davis gives us a gestural aesthetic that undoes the satisfactions of a narrative that would otherwise insult with resolution and reparativity, a happy ending–style merging of the desire for a center with anything deemed actual. Even negatively, in "Break It Down," she models an aspiration to loosen the storytelling we wrangle to be attached to the world, which involves reconceiving the objects/ scenes of the world as laboratories for an ongoing question of how living might be structured. The question remains ongoing and intractable; at the same time, that it is an ongoing question puts us in the realm of the predictables. That it is a question whose answer would not negate its persistence *as a question* puts us in the realm of the multiple actions and dynamics that change what a question, or negativity, can mean.

LE: There's a telling moment in "Break It Down" to which you made reference earlier. What matters about it to me in this context is how the force of a nonrelation erupts in response to an act of reading that both disturbs and promotes conversation:

> We were in bed and she asked me, Do I seem fat to you? and I was surprised because she didn't seem to worry about herself at all in that way and I guess I was reading into it that she did worry about herself so I answered what I was thinking and said stupidly that she had a very beautiful body, that her body was perfect, and I really meant it as an answer, but she said, kind of sharply, That's not what I asked, and so I had to try to answer her again, exactly what she had asked. (130)

Nothing in the story turns on this incident; it occasions no narrative consequence. Body size, beauty, the woman's self-perceptions: none of these emerge as thematic concerns anywhere else in the text. Instead this incident points to the structural impediment to relation that springs from the opacity of the otherness (whether internal or external to the subject) that induces relation in some sense to *situate* that opacity and contain it. When the woman, at least from the man's perspective, responds to him "kind of sharply," the edge of that sharpness leaves a troubling gash in the relational scene he has staged. But the gash itself then plays its part in his recalibration of the scene, responding in this not merely to local exigencies of understanding (leading to more or less rational revisions of earlier assumptions) but also to the specific imperative of his fundamental fantasy, which determines his place in the various scenarios he's capable of mobilizing.

Changes of scene, like changes of object, occur in this framework of attachment to a given structure of enjoyment. Neither changing the scene nor changing our objects can change our subjection to that framework or to the compulsion that drives those changes with the goal of *preserving* those attachments. The changes, the shifts in scene or language, transform the texture of experience by introducing new tropes, new representations of relational possibilities. But in doing so they merely define the figural repertoire of the subject, the particular set of fantasy scenes in which that subject can bear to play. To encounter this indistinguishability of change and repetition can make conversation, and the reading of the other on which it relies, a deeply demanding experience—and can make it, sometimes, more than that, which is to say, unbearable. For at any moment it can bring us to encounter the absolute limit of relation: the Real of nonrelation that relation contains, in more senses than one.

It's these multiple senses that words always carry and the particular valences they gain over time in the idiolects each of us speaks that make conversation a site of encounter with the impossibility of reading, no matter how close, no matter how patient one's practice of reading may be. Consider, as an instance of the problem, a series of sentences from our own conversation. Earlier you said of the second narrator that by "giving his story over, consciously or not, he opens the possibility of its crumbling in front of another— no longer in the trembling of sex, but in the expansive uncuratedness of conversation, a scene inevitably of nonsovereign relationality as such." Responding to this, I subsequently wrote, "Though I don't think conversation is 'inevitably' a 'scene . . . of nonsovereign relationality' (all too often—perhaps even in Davis's text—it becomes the fantasmatic scene of sovereign assertion), I do think it marks the site of a potential encounter with the unbearable: the otherness that permits no relation despite our best efforts to construct one." You began your last post by replying, "Conversation does require nonsovereignty, whether or not it feels otherwise or is marked manifestly by controlling gestures." I cite this conversation *about* conversation as exemplary of two points demonstrated *by* our conversation: first, that the encounter with an interlocutor shapes conversation as, among other things, a sequence of *missed* encounters; second, that you and I have managed, despite this, to locate the area in which our theoretical differences *can* find ways to bring something into being.

To make the first point clearer, let me note that between your original assertion and your reiteration of it in your last response, something crucial has dropped out. Initially you presented conversation as "inevitably" a "scene" of "nonsovereign relationality." Later the notion of the scene disappeared and conversation was said to "require nonsovereignty" in and of itself. In responding to your first formulation, it was this reference to a "scene" on which I picked up, since "scene," as you noted in your last response, invokes the setting of a fantasy. And precisely as a scene of fantasy, conversation, I argued, does *not* "inevitably" become a "scene . . . of nonsovereign relationality"; indeed it takes shape quite often as a scene of consolidating or asserting sovereignty, a scene that keeps the missed encounter from registering as such. That's why I offered a different formulation and described conversation as a "site," not a "scene": a site that bears the "potential" for an "encounter with the unbearable," with "nonsovereign relationality," and hence with the bar or barrier to relation, the nonrelation in relation itself.

When you return to the claim that conversation "does require nonsovereignty, whether or not it feels otherwise," I take it that you mean something similar to what I do when I call conversation a "site" (thereby focusing on the radical otherness in its structure that one may or may not encounter in any given conversation) rather than a "scene" (which would direct our attention, by contrast, to its fantasmatic frame). In drawing this distinction, I'm trying to determine if we're confronting a substantive intellectual disagreement or merely being sidetracked by each other's distinct linguistic scenes. For surely we both have noticed in the course of these conversations, and anyone encountering our dialogue must surely have noticed too, the different linguistic worlds we inhabit and the bearing of that difference on the political and theoretical scenes we produce. Theory, in its engagement with politics, must attend to the consequences of such differences, which produce the misses

in encounter, the mistakes we take for understandings in the tragi-
comedy of (non)relation.

The difference in thinking conversation as a site or a scene is not
"just" semantic; it can serve to epitomize our different ways of in-
flecting negativity. Who could deny that your version of negativity
feels more "livable" than mine? Your attention to "worlding" seeks
changes of scene that rescript the insistence of the unbearable, that
put it into motion and displace its pressure where it threatens to
crush the subject. I also maintain the importance of change but
focus on changing, on undoing, the subject rather than the subject's scene. For the scene's variations still manifest the subject's
fundamental fantasy—the fantasy that determines the range of
play the subject is able to bear, which is also to say, that the subject
can survive while remaining *fundamentally* the same. As such these
variations of scene can serve, among other things, as a screen to
keep what produces them unthought. But encountering what's truly
unbearable, attempting to push through the barrier of ourselves,
means approaching the limit of fantasy as the medium of desire
and finding ourselves in the movement of the drive that *structures*
our changes of scene. This is the movement around a real lack (the
gap of a primal negation) that might, as "The Center of the Story"
suggests, be construed in at least two ways: as the lack *of* a center
and the lack *at* the center, which, as Davis cannily writes, "is or is
not the same thing" (2010, 177).

If the object of desire, as I put it earlier, would "positivize" this
lack, it's not because I construe the object as "more homogeneous"
than you do; to the contrary, the object is always, for me, a fantasmatic placeholder (always exchangeable for others), an illusory
binding of contradictory pressures, possibilities, and investments
to defend the subject against the lack with which it can have no relation. That lack is what's unbearable, which is what I was saying
earlier, and what you misconstrued when you quoted me as saying
that "otherness . . . permits no relation despite our best efforts to
construct one." Though the words are mine, they've been stripped
from their context in which they describe "the unbearable," refer-
ring to it as "*the* otherness that permits no relation despite our best
efforts to construct one" (emphasis added). It's *that* otherness,

which I elsewhere describe as an "irreducible otherness," with which we can have no relation: the otherness of the lack or negativity that persists in undoing all positivization, in erupting as non-relation from within the fantasy of relationality.

The prospect of movement, in politics or in theory, derives from such unbearable encounters that break down the structuring fantasy of the subject. What follows from this is not living on but the prospect instead of living—where *living* means, for me as for you, living with negativity, experiencing a movement within contradiction, an identification with the force that would break down the barriers to the lack that breaks us down, or what Davis calls, in lines that you quote, "a part of you you have no control over." To break it down, where the subject is concerned, doesn't free it from determination by structure, repair its incoherence, or liberate it from fantasy. "Break It Down" remains an imperative: an imperative we can neither refuse to obey nor once and for all fulfill. But that imperative alone makes it possible, at the cost of encountering pain's metal bar, to have moments when living is neither survival nor merely postponement of death. That's why I wholly agree with your call for an "alternative orientation toward narrative." For neither of us does teleology offer political or theoretical promise. Instead, for both of us, it closes things down; it silences and immures.

But Davis supplants teleology with the ironies of consciousness. Her characters wrestle with whether they're reading the world or their own projections, with whether there ever could be for them a world *outside* their projections, with whether the selves they imagine are unreliable projections too. In the lines you quote from "How Shall I Mourn Them?" she asks, because she cannot know in advance, what form her incorporation of loss, inevitable as it is, will take: what sort of torsion she'll undergo without seeing it as such, without, that is, perceiving it as a form of mourning at all. The encounter with this lack of knowledge leaves the subject in a permanent state of emergency where the laws of identity are suspended and the rule of irony takes hold, establishing as absolute provision that all provisions be only provisional.

This rule of irony should not be confused with some particular form of affect—with a hip sensibility, a casual indifference, a privileged aloofness, a hard-boiled attitude, or any other mode of self-presentation. Instead such irony undermines every affirmative presentation of self and guarantees only the persistence, in its multitude of forms, of the negativity, the unresolved question, that drives us to pick at the scab of selfhood that aims to suture the wound of being. This is where, to borrow your phrase, I locate political potentiality, by which I mean the potential to experience the negativity that is the political: the division *within* community as well as the division *from* community; the division that leaves community, like the self, an always unresolved question. I'd like to think that you and I come together, in our different idiolects, in exploring the impulse, which I call the drive, to pursue this "ongoing question," the question whose very ongoingness bespeaks its negativity. We come together, that is, in our willingness to encounter the possibility of coming apart in the work and enjoyment of thinking that Davis theorizes in "Break It Down."

LB: Hmmm, fat, gashes, and scabs being picked at: the intensities of close reading cannot help but distort their object, inducing the irony to which you anchor negativity, but irony is not always uncanny or dramatic. When overattention and inattention merge (in love, in close reading's method, in friendship, there is no alternative), it's a little crazy and comic too, with all of the aggression and pleasure entailed. So, as I never suggested that anyone or any relation was freed, repaired, or liberated from anything by thinking about it, I do not know to what, or maybe whom, you're responding when you stake that claim. But our fantasy that a collaborative movement between us might be happening even here is not just a disavowal of our incapacity to achieve consistency or unambivalence. To stay in the situation involves remaining curious about how experimentality *must* involve the distortions of misrecognition on all sides, precisely because we are trying, together and separately, to induce a shift in what it means to be within the instability of the encounter.

In a related kind of contrast, the scene of nonsovereignty I was describing points to "the encounter" not just as a test of completion or repair but also as a scene in which one risks getting inside of a thing whose qualities will appear only in the action of its extension. This thing, this relation, this "it," taps into a prediction of the possibilities released by attunement. But what is attunement? In a sat-isfying conversation, attunement is not bound to having the same relation to content and prospects for world-building or narrative. These are archives and media for experiencing already established relations, in relation to which the process of encounter makes room for the interlocutors to emerge in their variousness, even when their needs for inattention and attention do not quite mesh and are not quite resolved. Those experiences from within collaborative ordi-nariness get us through the day, the week, the month, the world, life; they also shape, in the political register, the affective sense of justice, fairness, and recognition as more than formal acknowledg-ments.

Thus sex, activism, stranger encounters, reading—any collabo-rative practice—are not just performances of disavowal of the ob-ject's placeholderness but scenes of a drama of attention in which we seek to work out relationality, which is a task alongside of our aims to explain, maintain, and control the encounter. Most encoun-ters, anyway, sexual and otherwise, are forgettable and demand only minor attention; they rely on riding the efficiency of the norm. De-manding encounters, like paying attention to a lover, a friend, a col-league, worker, or disciplinary agent—anyone whose satisfaction matters—force us to confront how little we want to disturb our-selves within the scenes of attunement we also must of necessity seek. One flails around wanting something other than what is, but one also fears the disappointment of one's lack of imagination and trust in the patience and inventiveness of others.

But to me it's not *politics* if we are not trying to see how to change the consequences of what happens when the scene we are in shifts our orientation in ways we do not control. To me, it's politics if we are seeking to change the consequences and resonances of the appearance of the foundational antagonisms. Your story is about facing how persons are controlled by those ways and their aims to deny them, and my story is that as we move with each other, when we can, we can shift the consequences of what's irreparable and out of joint in our internal and social relations. We don't *necessarily* shift them, but this is what it means to do our work collectively. Because of our curiosity about how it will work out (will it be broken down or transformed?), because of our desires not to be defeated by life, we enter the scene of relationality that is also and ultimately a demand for collaboration; relationality disturbs fantasy enough that it is open to crazy controls and also to absorbing and generating new social relations.

Maybe you believe less in the structural generativity of this worlding work than I do; I don't know. I do know that central to my own approach to this conversation has been not to take on many of your challenges directly in order not endlessly to dig into our positions under the fantasy that in so doing either of us will persuade the other. To me, the great pleasure of any collaboration is multiplying idioms and infrastructures for further thought that neither of us could have generated alone. If not repair, what? If not worldbuilding, what? If the inevitable nonencounter, then what? Working with aesthetic exempla has been our way of further extending that practice, reading with our objects as allies in a double collaboration aimed toward discovering why it is that we address unbearable out-of-jointness so similarly and yet with such different anxieties about what occupying a structure entails.

What would you do if I closed by saying, Okay, you win, you're right: the capacity to make new settings for occupying the irreparable rivenness of subjects and worlds is just my fantasy of the possibility of social and personal transformation, and in the end really is merely reparative, really is just trying to distract me from the ways it's unbearable to be partnered by one's brokenness and saturated by the bad, wearing world? What would you do if I acted like the narrator and responded dutifully and dissociatively to the question "Do you think I'm fat?" I don't think you'd feel satisfied. Would you dance around the house, pumping your fists in the air? No, I don't think you would.

Were I to take on your view it would feel as if I'd withdrawn from the ethics of the conversation, which is to maintain fidelity to the question cluster we've developed over time, even as we face, in our own ways, the loneliness and the gash of the failed encounter around those questions. So we made a context for the work in a register that is not bound precisely to the terms that we're debating. This way, although we have not resolved how best to live with or even think about negativity, we've opened up for ourselves—and we hope for our readers—some clarity about what is at stake in the debate over nonsovereign subjectivity and its vicissitudes in sex, theory, aesthetics, politics, fantasy, and attachment. We have seen described and enacted some of the kinds of violence done in the name of fantasy, of disavowing the impossibility of repairing relationality simply. We have debated whether it matters what tone we take toward the recognition of the work of the structural. And we have seen that there is pleasure in working it out together, for example, in worlding practices.

In this mode of attention toward attunement, there is no romance to the work of theory and no repair through the work of romance. There is converging that is inseparable from abandonment, movement within varieties of intense stuckness, and foreclosing gestures that are also openings, because we are thinking together and with other things and thinkers. The work of theory and of sexual normativity cannot be said to resolve any problem related to the inevitable violence of the nonencounter with ourselves and the world. But the drive to inhabit what passes among intimates and strangers and publics is another sense in which to "break it down" is to make an "it" happen that is predicated on our desires for the nonsovereign and the relational without predication.

Sometimes the struggle to attend to this without foreclosure is difficult, but the desire for "it" is not merely unbearable and taken care of by the irony that stages in language the ruination of the fantasy of repair. Alongside of what's hard, as all of our cases have shown, are examples of the unbearable question that point us to a different understanding of structure not as noun but as verb, as embedded in the gestures we make to make radiant exempla, things into scene, and the struggle, which is collective before it is mutual, to make new terms for the encounter that restages the desire for attachment alongside all of the ways that we fight it.

LE: As this conversation has surely made clear, my mode of being present to it is to "take on many of your challenges directly," to respond to the specific language and form you give to your ideas. And I do so "under the fantasy" you explicitly reject: "that either of us will persuade the other." That doesn't mean, on the one hand, that I consciously invest in some notion of "winning," as in an argument or a quarrel; we approached this conversation from the outset not as a debate but as a *dialogue* about the place of negativity in political projects we both conceive as inseparable from theory, narrative, and sex. But it doesn't mean, on the other hand, that we escape the *fantasy* of persuasion either: not a persuasion that would be global (surrender-inducing, once and for all), but one that allows us to recognize when the other has shown that a particular claim, or the form of its assertion, needs adjustment or isn't stable in the way that it's been framed. Such a possibility of being persuaded that something other than what we recognize may bear on and valuably change the shape of our original understandings derives from our common commitment, first and foremost, to ideas and to the enjoyment to be found in their continuous reencounter and modification. That's what makes our conversation, to my way of thinking, collaborative. Like any form of pedagogy, it operates at the uncertain border where persuasion and seduction meet. Except as a rhetorical gesture, therefore, we can't renounce persuasion. But that doesn't make agreement the point toward which we ought to tend.

In the give-and-take of dialogue, our primal attachments may lead us from one mode of analysis to another, from one example to another, from one form of argument to another, in a metonymic movement that never abandons those attachments even as we respond to the other's critical and theoretical claims. This movement, reflecting the gap that reopens on every approach to "it," accounts for what I've been calling the impossibility of encounter: the impossibility, more precisely, of encountering the nonsovereignty exemplified by the drive. That's why I describe this impossible encounter as properly unbearable. It's impossible *because* unbearable for the subject *as subject of fantasy.* And that's why sex, which always takes place in proximity to the unbearable, can also, in the realm of Panoptimism, aspire to *take its place,* to repair the ruptures of negativity by *realizing* relation, as if sex might be able to positivize it, literally to flesh it out. That doesn't, of course, mean that sex is always a positive experience, only that it's often expected to produce the sort of positivization by means of which otherness is accommodated, relation made material, and negativity overcome.

But relation's materiality lies neither in the flesh nor in our positivizations of it; it lies instead in the signifying system within which it appears. As a consequence, sex emerges as tragicomic conversation, as a mode of exchange or a form of intercourse that *Me and You and Everyone We Know* invokes by way of its logo:)) < > ((. The lozenge (< >), the "poop," that passes from one set of buttocks to the other in the logo, oblivious to particularizing differences such as gender, race, or age, and erasing the legibility of active and passive positions in sex, remains forever suspended, as if affirming the "inter" of intercourse and figuring what joins and separates subjects who form (and are formed by) inverted brackets that contain and totalize nothing. Exchange takes place through a signifier here that would signify exchange as such: a signifier capable of transmuting shit into meaning as relationality. Ultimately, though, that relation itself is a relation *to* the signifier and all the divisions that determine it, divisions that keep us (as the logo and Davis's story both suggest) always at a distance from "sex," from "it," from radical encounter with the other, which is *other than signification*. The impossibility that structures the encounter, however, doesn't make relation impossible; as relation depends on negativity, so negativity constitutes relation. But that relation can never be positivized; we can never know in what it consists or with whom or what it's played out. Instead, as the logo demonstrates, it exists in the form of continuous exchange, in the openness of (and to) our questioning the forms of its possibility.

This, for me, is what's at stake in the negativity of politics. You write, "To me it's not *politics* if we are not trying to see how to change the consequences of what happens when the scene we are in shifts our orientation in ways we do not control." But we can't control or predict in advance what consequences (for us or for anyone else) will follow from a change in our orientation that's defined as beyond our control. The change that politics makes lies rather in keeping the question of relation (to oneself, to others, and therefore to politics) open to the negativity with which relation is bound up—and open, therefore, to the irony of attempts to totalize politics or community by negating those who embody its negativity, its "antisociality."

You say that if you were to "take on my view" it would constitute a withdrawal from the ethics that have guided our conversation. I agree with you completely. Having you adopt "my view" and so end the movement of our conversation has never been my goal. Flourishing demands the conversation itself, the open-endedness (as the logo depicts it) by which, as in Johnson's Untitled (Ass), enjoyment can find its occasion in what might seem to erase us as well. The shaping of our claims in terms of various rhetorics of persuasion thus solicits, in this context, resistance, counterargument, and the teasing out of thought that allows us both to rework our ideas as they pass through the filter of the other. Would I pump my fist in triumph should you accede to my positions? Not at all. But I'd love to be persuaded by you; I'd love to be able to believe that "as we move with each other, when we can, we can shift the consequences of what's irreparable and out of joint in our internal and social relations." It's because I'm drawn to and admire your vision of "moving with the unbearable," as I admire and am drawn to Leo Bersani's attempts to think what "play[s] to the side of" jouissance without, in the process, denying it, that I want to keep this conversation alive and put pressure on your reading of the irreparable (2010, 65). I want to believe, for example, as you say in chapter 1, that acknowledging and dedramatizing negativity could produce a context in which "the virtue squad [would] not be able to use dramas of threatened sexual security to reproduce the normative good life." But I don't, as yet, see proof that we can shift the *consequences* of the irreparable. What else, after all, are those consequences but the endless movements of negativity, with all the violence that comes from our various ways of enacting and denying it? But also, therefore, with all the possibility of dissent from totalizing norms. Those consequences, in short, include *politics as negativity's expression*. And that, for me, is why fighting our own misrecognitions matters, even if misrecognition as such remains, in the end, inevitable. Such resistance defines the work of thought as a movement, not an end, as an endless self-undoing whose negativity brings us to life. Challenging the fixity of "me" and "you" and "everyone we know," this conversation enacts that negativity for me and remains, as a consequence, intimate, political, open-ended, and imperative: a fragment of our ongoing efforts to encounter what's other, to break "it" down.

LB: The hardest thing for me in this conversation has been to listen well to you, responding to your account of the subject's and the world's dialectic of intractable negativity, while also exploring my own interest in how things multiply, are overdetermined, and move in relation nonetheless. We were brought together as like-minded polemicists against futurity. Your argument against the optimism in futurity was that it enables the straight-identified world to disavow the unbearable fact that it will never coincide with itself and never really reproduce itself, except insofar as it projects out fantasies of repair through the subordination of disturbing enemies, like queers. For me, the problem of futurity's perspective is in the presumption that *contemporary* structural subordinations are intractable. I insist instead on a less austere materialism of a continuously contemporary ordinariness, in which beings try to make do and to flourish in the awkward, riven, unequal, untimely, and interesting world of other beings, abstractions, and forces, and in which we therefore have a shot at transforming the dynamics and the costs of our negativity and its appearance. So many different kinds of structure organize the estrangements and attachments of the world that how we are to live among and transform their existence both materially and in fantasy is my central question. Antifuturism for me therefore shapes the terms of urgency and curiosity through which we make worlds for transforming life now. Politics, like affect, and like theory, has to attend to the present that it is also generating.

But our focus has moved on too, from the question of futurity to that of collaboration as a figure of relation. We did not predict this. In sex, in politics, in theory—in any infrastructure that we can call intimate or invested with the activity of living—we cannot banish the strangeness in ourselves or of anything in the world. While we can point to the impossibility of staying reliable to one's self- and other-directed relations and to the impact of the ways we fail them, though, these contacts can spark new forms of life, of being in the scene of relationality, whose effects are always being calculated yet are beyond calculation. Even though I can imagine agreeing to an account of politics "as negativity's expression," I am stymied to think what kinds of argument and evidence you would have to encounter not to see the transformative force of recontextualization since you practice it yourself. But bafflement is an integral part of the pleasure and sometimes the comedy of the intimate, just as disbelief is a core affect of the political.

In this book, for me, the opening up of the encounter between negativity and nonsovereignty has been the great revelation of sex in its various forms. Sex and love are not events that change anything, usually; they induce a loosening of the subject that puts fear, pleasure, awkwardness, and above all experimentality in a scene that forces its participants to disturb what it has meant to be a person and to "have" a world. It forces people to *desire* to be nonsovereign, and sometimes not-autonomous, and that puts them in intimate proximity to play, aversion, and unbearable intensity. When it takes the shape of intimate relationality, it is both disturbing and anchoring, and therefore never stilled enough to be a concrete foundation for the house of life or the house of pain; expressing a desire for disturbance, sex cannot also defend entirely against it. But when put in proximity to pleasure, the unbearable is also borne, and the riven accompanied by banality and varieties of attunement. It breaks us down in multiple, nonidentical ways, all of which are in a complex relation to the fantasy of relation itself.

As all of our chapters demonstrate, and as "Break It Down" stages so brilliantly, the impact of any encounter cannot just involve an estimate of whether it was "worth it," successful, or added up to something, as though the dominant register of the calculation is the only register possible. This is what it means to live, and to theorize, experimentally: to make registers of attention and assessment that can change the world of their implication, but also to model the suspension of knowing in a way that dilates attention to a problem or scene. This involves the pain and pleasure of unlearning or "breaking down" what we thought our object was and who we are in relation to it; this involves moving with it without assurance of what we might become as we refuse to reproduce the lines of association, convergence, and force whose security defended us from the disturbance that, we say, we also want. In the meanwhile, the pursuit of clarifying and transformative phrases, exempla, and archives holds up the world with which we are inevitably, sometimes happily, and always fantasmatically, in relation. "And it's still all a surprise and it never stops, even after it's over, it never stops being a surprise" (128).

AFTERWORDS

We close this book with two afterwords. Given our interest in shifting the available genres of theoretical encounter, we wanted these afterwords to break from both the collective voice of the preface and the dialogic responsiveness of the chapters themselves. So we decided to write our afterwords separately, unaware of what the other would say or what form that saying would take. We hoped to discover what we each had learned from our collaborative work on this project and to look back at our exchanges while answering the loaded question, How was it for you?

Unsurprisingly, no reader could wonder for a moment which afterword was written by whom. For better or worse, our voices, in all their differences, come through loud and clear. But what does surprise us, given the argument foregrounded throughout this text, is how close we come to each other in certain crucial formulations, especially where we both converge on the pedagogy of surprise. Insofar as critical practice takes shape as an intimate encounter—with one's own ideas, with an object's otherness, with the voices of countless scholars—we do not intend these afterwords as the last word in any way. Nor do we think our conversation, or the effect of our having had it, is over. As the man accounting for his sexual adventure in "Break It Down" insists, "It isn't over when it ends, it goes on after it's all over" (129). That's what an intimate encounter means and what we mean by the encounter that animates us in *Sex, or the Unbearable*.

It Isn't Over

It seems fitting that our final chapter ends on the word "surprise." With its etymological link to being seized, overtaken, or taken over, *surprise* defines the encounter with what disrupts our expectations by breaking through the defensive barriers associated with routine. To that extent surprise inheres in experiences of nonsovereignty that take us (as, for example, in sex) beyond our familiar limits—if only, as so often with sex, in largely familiar ways. Even those subjects who live with the expectation of nonsovereignty (children and prisoners, among others) can find a vestige of sovereignty in that very expectation, thus normalizing those limits into the logic of a world. It takes a lot of attention and a willingness to be seized by something one cannot know in advance to retain the capacity for surprise before what offers itself as what is; it takes a continuous resistance to one's englobement by "the world."

The paradigmatic form of such resistance is the drive. In contrast to the investment in fantasy that vivifies desire, affirming a world where objects have the power to complete us, the drive dismisses both objects and the aim of achieving completion. Enacting a negativity with no other end but its own insistence, the drive expresses the nonsovereignty brought home in what we've called "the encounter." Though the effects it generates constantly change, the negativity of the drive does not. Nor can it, properly speaking, be taken as an object of desire. No wonder negativity gets such bad press. It shrinks from positivization in any program of political action and undermines whatever we take as an a priori good. Like the drive, that is, it affirms no good beyond its own persistence: the good (but is it a good at all?—negativity can never affirm it) of encounter, interruption, disturbance, unmaking, disappropriation, subtraction, surprise.

But surprise is often unpleasant. The jolt it induces, the shock of what we didn't or couldn't anticipate, reminds us that whatever the feelings a given instance of it inspires, surprise corresponds to a breach of security and so to a possible threat. Another name for that threat, as this book has argued, might be life, where life entails vulnerability to the unpredictable encounter that can often seem, with regard to the selves that we recognize, unbearable. Who wants destabilization when what's destabilized is us, our place in the world, our deepest values, the political goals we advance? Shouldn't negativity shake the ground our political rivals stand on without its seismic ripples causing us to topple too? But the encounter buffets the world as it is and us in a single blow. How could it ever do otherwise when we are the products of that world? We claim that we want to break it down, but our wanting, our desire as subjects (insofar as we view that desire *as ours*), no more survives the encounter intact than does the subject itself. Negativity-lite is no option.

That explains why these dialogues, in the process of thinking the conditions for change, keep coming back to the unbearable in the encounter with negativity. Negativity is unchanging *as structure* because negativity *structures change*. Far from being incompatible, structure and change are inextricable. In any given instance, though, we need to ask some questions to understand their relation more fully: What sort of change are we talking about? What level of structure do we aim to describe? What scale of attention do we deploy to distinguish between change and repetition? It might, for example, seem surprising to some that this book, in which we explicitly advocate openness to surprise, should "keep coming back to the . . . unbearable" as if to iterations of the same. That the embedding of surprise in repetition is able repeatedly to surprise us speaks to the incessant pressure of what we continue not to know. But our coming back to the unbearable is never just a return to the same. What's unbearable in negativity is its vertiginous nonidentity, the disunity we fail to comprehend however much we think we know our own and the world's incoherence. Our encounters with negativity, like the repetitions of the drive, may change our objects, ourselves, and our relation to what surrounds us. They may alter our experience of being in the world in ways both large and small. But they do so without, for all of that, affecting the persistence of the unbearable or the force of its structural consequences, including the urge to negate whatever contingently (and therefore variably) may figure its negativity.

All of which serves to remind us of what we far prefer to forget: the unbearable names what cannot be borne by the subjects we think we are. We build our worlds in the face of it so as to keep ourselves *from* facing it, as if we implicitly understood that the unbearable as such can have no face and works to deprive us of ours. Though meant to forestall the unbearable, such world-building no more escapes it than do our attempts at political change. But the fact of that structural imperative discredits neither world-building nor political struggle; to the contrary, it interprets such struggle itself as integral to negativity's structure. It suggests, moreover, that politics derives from a negativity indifferent to the future, a negativity that insists, in the present tense, on the urgency of politics as the ceaseless drive of resistance and dissent. One might even add: for their own sake, which is also to say, for ours.

Exploring how negativity casts off its every reification, including attempts to oppose it simplistically to optimism, sociality, or repair, these conversations have tried to be true to negativity's creative destruction, enacting the otherness of relation as seen in the moment of encounter. Perhaps, then, the most surprising thing about *Sex, or the Unbearable* is its suggestion that the word we understand least in its title may be "or."

—LEE EDELMAN

After It's Over

At one difficult time during the writing of this book, after a heated phone call about where our work was headed, I returned to the text to respond to what I felt was some misreading of the grounding of my arguments. In that writing, as often, I was feeling my way, both focused on moving the discussion forward (about what it means to seek to transform what's nonsovereign in desire and unbearable in relation) and also irritated about how I'd been characterized. Yet I also did not want to become stubborn and stentorian, pulling our work off-track by making it about me rather than the problem at hand, which I hoped wasn't me! But in collaboration, as in love, or even ordinary conversation, one can never be sure.

I began writing with a digression from our shared focus on the impossibility of repairing, mastering, or even being adequate to the intimate encounter and turned instead to the James Mason film *Bigger than Life* (Ray 1956). *Bigger than Life* is about an English teacher after World War II who is rescued from a heart problem by a new miracle drug, steroids. But, as both Lee and I would predict, the repair also injures, transforming the story of cause and effect to a spectacle of cause and side effects. Steroids make Mason a hyper-masculine sadist, inflated with sexual and intellectual grandiosity and seething with contempt at the pathetic self-esteem obsessions of the bourgeois parents whose children he teaches. At the same time he oscillates in his affect, weeping and overwhelmed by the appearance through him of an aggression he cannot fully own as his. Then, paradoxically and spontaneously, he seethes at his own wife and child for their weakness, their own refusal to be Bigger than Life like him, and their resistance to the rules he has set up to enable a superior askesis, or discipline of life.

In one scene, Mason, with his enormous head, is helping his small, soft son to do his math homework. Helping turns to intimidation and bullying. As the scene intensifies and becomes scary, the son gets worse at the math that he already cannot do. They are trying to parse a story problem. As an exercise in the assessment and force of relation, the story problem often finds its way into the narration of love. (Lover X does this, and lover Y does that: Why, then, is the outcome Z?) Here, to find a common denominator, the child adds six and five when the task warrants multiplying. He gets the conjunctures of relation wrong. The father's critical voice deepens and the son's defensive voice gets higher. As the voices intensify, the commanding voice penetrates the room and siphons the child's

FIG A.1. Love, teaching, intimacy . . . or the unbearable. *Bigger Than Life* (1956).

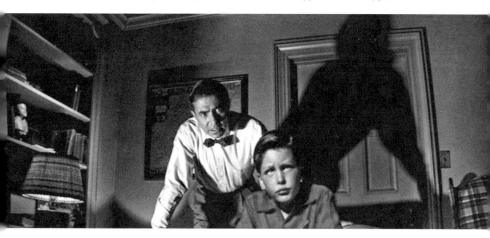

confidence. Then the father behind the desk crosses over to the son at the table, as though his physical proximity will produce a greater clarity of thought. This shift converts the wall into a screen, as the silhouette of the dominating father towers over his cowering son (figure A.1).

This dumb show *in nuce*, this shadow puppet show, is haunting and terrifying. It is as though the film turns at once toward affective inflation and a demonstration of the magic of cinema in order to distract the audience from the pure brutality it also continues to demonstrate. Even when it is crowded out by other gestures of enabling and gifting, even when turning toward and turning away from our objects is executed with good intentions, this tableau of a bullying pedagogy is desperately ordinary at the heart of love.

I was surprised to be writing about *Bigger Than Life* as though Lee had cast me as the woman or the child in that film, appearing in these pages variously as the weak theorist, the reparative sociologist, the politically correct subject seeking out the virtuous archive and reparative gesture, the reader who missed a crucial point. True enough! But was I so sure that I did not want to dominate Lee back through some kind of lateral-minded sweetness or a Nietzschean weak-strong countertheorizing style? My question opened onto the vista of contradictory desires that intimate encounters *will* animate: to dominate; not to dominate; to avoid being dominated; to submit to his claim so as to get on with things, or to give in to a partial agreement; to listen hard to find what's movable in the situation; to give as good as I get; to be equal; to try both to get it rightish conceptually *and* between us. Then I started laughing at what a perfect scene this crazy condensation in *Bigger Than Life* was for demonstrating the cluster of impossible and unbearable interests we bring to relationality—in this book, *Sex, or the Unbearable*, I mean.

So, sheepishly, in our next phone call, I told Lee of this outtake I had written and what I had learned from writing it, and it turned out that, lo, he too had memorized *Bigger than Life*, or been dented by it, and the same scenes and the same problems, without exactly identifying all over it (and there we are, not identical). We started laughing and riffing all over the place, drawing from the kinds of things we know (more psychoanalytic, in his case; more materialist and affective in mine; aesthetically focused for both of us) to make some sense of the impact of this film. This kind of open ferocity and friendliness was exemplary of the collaborative spirit that made this book possible for us and enabled us to be educated by the process of writing it, even when our encounters radically diverged or just shifted awkwardly in the ballpark of a mutual clarification. But of course I would claim this, since the position I hold in what you've just read is that making a world for what doesn't work changes the consequences of those failures in a way that produces new potentials for relation within the structural space of the nonsovereign.

I might rest my case by being my final case. Throughout the book, though, there is no finishing off of the structural problems with an optimistic inversion, comic displacement, capstone phrase, or decisive vignette. There is no formula—no form—that can anchor the *or* that marks the problem our title poses. Sex, collaboration, and relationality as such require us to learn to walk in the wet sand of the questions that shift on the occasion of an impact by another, even when that impact involves something as small as another's phrasing. Why should our critical work be different from any other object whose force affects what it seems possible to think, to do, and to undo?

I do not read things; I read with things. When I read with theorists, with art, with a colleague or a friend, *to read with* is to cultivate a quality of attention to the disturbance of their alien epistemology, an experience of nonsovereignty that shakes my confidence in a way from which I have learned to derive pleasure, induce attachment, and maintain curiosity about the enigmas and insecurities that I can also barely stand or comprehend. This is what it means to say that excitement is disturbing, not devastating; ambivalent, not shattering in the extreme. Structural consistency is a fantasy; the noise of relation's impact, inducing incompletion where it emerges, is the overwhelming condition that enables the change that, within collaborative action, can shift lived worlds.

—LAUREN BERLANT

Break It Down

LYDIA DAVIS

He's sitting there staring at a piece of paper in front of him. He's trying to break it down. He says:

I'm breaking it all down. The ticket was $600 and then after that there was more for the hotel and food and so on, for just ten days. Say $80 a day, no, more like $100 a day. And we made love, say, once a day on the average. That's $100 a shot. And each time it lasted maybe two or three hours so that would be anywhere from $33 to $50 an hour, which is expensive.

Though of course that wasn't all that went on, because we were together almost all day long. She would keep looking at me and every time she looked at me it was worth something, and she smiled at me and didn't stop talking and singing, something I said, she would sail into it, a snatch, for me, she would be gone from me a little ways but smiling too, and tell me jokes, and I loved it but didn't exactly know what to do about it and just smiled back at her and felt slow next to her, just not quick enough. So she talked and touched me on the shoulder and the arm, she kept touching and stayed close to me. You're with each other all day long and it keeps happening, the touches and smiles, and it adds up, it builds up, and you know where you'll be that night, you're talking and every now and then you think about it, no, you don't think, you just feel it as a kind of destination, what's coming up after you leave wherever you are all evening, and you're happy about it and you're planning it all, not in your head, really, somewhere inside your body, or all through your body, it's all mounting up and coming together so that when you get in bed you can't help it, it's a real performance, it all pours out, but slowly, you go easy until you can't anymore, or you hold back the whole time, you hold back and touch the edges of everything, you edge around until you have to plunge in and finish it off, and when you're finished, you're too weak to stand but after a while you have to go to the bathroom and you stand, your legs are trembling, you hold on to the door frames, there's a little light coming in through the window, you can see your way in and out, but you can't really see the bed.

So it's not really $100 a shot because it goes on all day, from the start when you wake up and feel her body next to you, and you don't miss a thing, not a thing of what's next to you, her arm, her leg, her shoulder, her face, that good skin, I have felt other good skin, but this skin is just the edge of something else, and you're going to start going, and no matter how much you crawl all over each other it won't be enough, and when your hunger dies down a little then you think how much you love her and that starts you off again, and her face, you look over at her face and can't believe how you got there and how lucky and it's still all a surprise and it never stops, even after it's over, it never stops being a surprise.

It's more like you have a good sixteen or eighteen hours a day of this going on, even when you're not with her it's going on, it's good to be away because it's going to be so good to go back to her, so it's still here, and you can't go off and look at some old street or some old painting without still feeling it in your body and a few things that happened the day before that don't mean much by themselves or wouldn't mean much if you weren't having this thing together, but you can't forget and it's all inside you all the time, so that's more like, say, sixteen into a hundred would be $6 an hour, which isn't too much.

And then it really keeps going on while you're asleep, though you're probably dreaming about something else, a building, maybe, I kept dreaming, every night, almost, about this building, because I would spend a lot of every morning in this old stone building and when I closed my eyes I would see these cool spaces and have this peace inside me, I would see the bricks of the floor and the stone arches and the space, the emptiness between, like a kind of dark frame around what I could see beyond, a garden, and this space was like a stone too because of the coolness of it and the gray shadow, that kind of luminous shade, that was glowing with the light of the sun falling beyond the arches, and there was also the great height of the ceiling, all this was in my mind all the time though I didn't know it until I closed my eyes, I'm asleep and I'm not dreaming about her but she's lying next to me and I wake up enough times in the night to remember she's there, and notice, say, once she was lying on her back but now she's curled around me, I look at her closed eyes, I want to kiss her eyelids, I want to feel that soft skin under my lips, but I don't want to disturb her, I don't want to see her frown as though in her sleep she has forgotten who I am and feels just that something is bothering her and so I just look at her and hold on to it all, these times when I'm watching over her sleep and she's next to me and isn't away from me the way she will be later, I want to stay awake all night just to go on feeling that, but I can't, I fall asleep again, though I'm sleeping lightly, still trying to hold on to it.

But it isn't over when it ends, it goes on after it's all over, she's still inside you like a sweet liquor, you are filled with her, everything about her has kind of bled into you, her smell, her voice, the way her body moves, it's all inside you, at least for a while after, then you begin to lose it, and I'm beginning to lose it, you're afraid of how weak you are, that you can't get her all back into you again and now the whole thing is going out of your body and it's more in your mind than your body, the pictures come to you one by one and you look at them, some of them last longer than others, you were together in a very white clean place, a coffeehouse, having breakfast together, and the place is so white that against it you can see her clearly, her blue eyes, her smile, the colors of her clothes, even the print of the newspaper she's reading when she's not looking up at you, the light brown and red and gold of her hair when she's got her head down reading, the brown coffee, the brown rolls, all against that white table and those white plates and silver urns and silver knives and spoons, and against that quiet of the sleepy people in that room sitting alone at their tables with just some chinking and clattering of spoons and cups in saucers and some hushed voices her voice now and then rising and falling. The pictures come to you and you have to hope they won't lose their life too fast and dry up though you know they will and that you'll also forget some of what happened, because already you're turning up little things that you nearly forgot.

We were in bed and she asked me, Do I seem fat to you? and I was surprised because she didn't seem to worry about herself at all in that way and I guess I was reading into it that she did worry about herself so I answered what I was thinking and said stupidly that she had a very beautiful body, that her body was perfect, and I really meant it as an answer, but she said kind of sharply, That's not what I asked, and so I had to try to answer her again, exactly what she had asked.

And once she lay over against me late in the night and she started talking, her breath in my ear, and she just went on and on, and talked faster and faster, she couldn't stop, and I loved it, I just felt that all that life in her was running into me too, I had so little life in me, her life, her fire, was coming into me, in that hot breath in my ear, and I just wanted her to go on talking forever right there next to me, and I would go on living, like that, I would be able to go on living, like that, I would be able to go on living, but without her I don't know.

Then you forget some of it all, maybe most of it all, almost all of it, in the end, and you work hard at remembering everything now so you won't ever forget, but you can kill it too even by thinking about it too much, though you can't help thinking about it nearly all the time.

And then when the pictures start to go you start asking some questions, just little questions, that sit in your mind without any answers, like why did she have the light on when you came in to bed one night, but it was off the next but she had it on the night after that and she had it off the last night, why, and other questions, little questions that nag at you like that.

And finally the pictures go and these dry little questions just sit there without any answers and you're left with this large heavy pain in you that you try to numb by reading, or you try to ease it by getting out into public places where there will be people around you, but no matter how good you are at pushing that pain away, just when you think you're going to be all right for awhile, that you're safe, you're kind of holding it off with all your strength and you're staying in some little bare numb spot of ground, then suddenly it will all come back, you'll hear a noise, maybe it's a cat crying or a baby, or something else like her cry, you hear it and make that connection in a part of you you have no control over and the pain comes back so hard that you're afraid, afraid of how you're falling back into it again, and you wonder, no, you're terrified to ask how you're ever going to climb out of it.

And so it's not only every hour of the day while it's happening, but it's really for hours and hours every day after that, for weeks, though less and less, so that you could work out the ratio if you wanted, maybe after six weeks you're only thinking about it an hour or so in the day altogether, a few minutes here and there spread over, or a few minutes here and there and half an hour before you go to sleep, or sometimes it all comes back and you stay awake with it half the night.

So when you add up all that, you've only spent maybe $3 an hour on it.

If you have to figure in the bad times too, I don't know. There weren't any bad times with her, though maybe there was one bad time, when I told her I loved her. I couldn't help it, this was the first time this had happened with her, now I was half falling in love with her or maybe completely if she had let me but she couldn't or I couldn't completely because it was all going to be so short and other things too, and so I told her, and didn't know of any way to tell her first that she didn't have to feel this was a burden, the fact that I loved her, or that she didn't have to feel the same about me, or say the same back, that it was just that I had to tell her, that's all, because it was bursting inside me, and saying it wouldn't even begin to take care of what I was feeling, really I couldn't say anything of what I was feeling because there was so much, words couldn't handle it, and making love only made it worse because then I wanted words badly but they were no good, no good at all, but I told her anyway, I was lying on top of her and her hands were up by her head and my hands were on hers and our fingers were locked and there was a little light on her face from the window but I couldn't really see her and I was afraid to say it but I had to say it because I wanted her to know, it was the last night, I had to tell her then or I'd never have another chance, I just said, Before you go to sleep, I have to tell you before you go to sleep that I love you, and immediately, right away after, she said, I love you too, and it sounded to me as if she didn't mean it, a little flat, but then it usually sounds a little flat when someone says, I love you too, because they're just saying it back even if they do mean it, and the problem is that I'll never know if she meant it, or maybe someday she'll tell me whether she meant it or not, but there's no way to know now, and I'm sorry I did that, it was a trap I didn't mean to put her in, I can see it was a trap, because if she hadn't said anything at all I know that would have hurt too, as though she were taking something from me and just accepting it and not giving anything back, so she really had to, even just to be kind to me, she had to say it, and I don't really know now if she meant it.

Another bad time, or it wasn't exactly bad, but it wasn't easy either, was when I had to leave, the time was coming, and I was beginning to tremble and feel empty, nothing in the middle of me, nothing inside, and nothing to hold me up on my legs, and then it came, everything was ready, and I had to go, and so it was just a kiss, a quick one, as though we were afraid of what might happen after a kiss, and she was almost wild then, she reached up to a hook by the door and took an old shirt, a green and blue shirt from the hook, and put it in my arms, for me to take away, the soft cloth was full of her smell, and then we stood there close together looking at a piece of paper she had in her hand and I didn't lose any of it, I was holding it tight, that last minute or two, because this was it, we'd come to the end of it, things always change, so this was really it, over.

Maybe it works out all right, maybe you haven't lost for doing it, I don't know, no, really, sometimes when you think of it you feel like a prince really, you feel just like a king, and then other times you're afraid, you're afraid, not all the time but now and then, of what it's going to do to you, and it's hard to know what to do with it now.

Walking away I looked back once and the door was still open, I could see her standing far back in the dark of the room, I could only really see her white face still looking out at me, and her white arms.

I guess you get to a point where you look at that pain as if it were there in front of you three feet away lying in a box, an open box, in a window somewhere. It's hard and cold, like a bar of metal. You just look at it there and say, All right, I'll take it, I'll buy it. That's what it is. Because you know all about it before you even go into this thing. You know the pain is part of the whole thing. And it isn't that you can say afterwards the pleasure was greater than the pain and that's why you would do it again. That has nothing to do with it. You can't measure it, because the pain comes after and it lasts longer. So the question really is, Why doesn't that pain make you say, I won't do it again? When the pain is so bad that you have to say that, but you don't.

So I'm just thinking about it, how you can go in with $600, more like $1,000, and how you can come out with an old shirt.

ACKNOWLEDGMENTS

We are fortunate to have had the support and assistance of many people who encouraged and made possible the production of this book. In the first place, we want to thank Heather Love. There would have been no book at all had Heather not invited us to speak at the conference she organized at the University of Pennsylvania in honor of Gayle Rubin. More than simply extending that initial invitation, however, Heather also responded enthusiastically to the joint paper we proposed and, in conversations afterward, suggested we turn it into a book. For that we are deeply grateful. We also extend sincere thanks to Michael Cobb for inviting us, on behalf of the Division on Literary Criticism, to participate on a panel at the MLA in memory of Eve Kosofsky Sedgwick, and to Elaine Freedgood for inviting us to present a segment of the chapter on "Break It Down" at a conference at New York University. These timely invitations helped shape the final form of this book and the audiences at those events provided important feedback and encouragement.

This book would have suffered greatly were it not for the assistance of two of the artists whose works we discuss within it. We are profoundly grateful to Larry Johnson for his friendliness and generosity in allowing us to reprint his color photograph Untitled (Ass). Both Stuart Krimko, of the David Kordansky Gallery in Los Angeles, and Russell Ferguson offered invaluable assistance in making our use of this photograph possible and we wish to take this opportunity to thank them for all their help. It is with genuine pleasure that we acknowledge our indebtedness to Lydia Davis for her remarkable support of our efforts to include the text of her story, "Break It Down," as an appendix to this book. Permission to reprint was

ACKNOWLEDGMENTS

facilitated by Babe Liberson and Hayley Davidson, whose efforts we greatly appreciate. We wish to thank Farrar, Straus and Giroux, LLC, and Penguin Books, Ltd., for granting us permission to reprint the text of "Break It Down." The negotiations for the rights to do so, like so many other crucial aspects of this book, were handled by Jade Brooks at Duke University Press. Her constant resourcefulness, her rapidity of response, and her endless and good-humored patience are just a few of the qualities for which we owe her more than these words can sufficiently indicate. Ken Wissoker has been an ideal editor at Duke; kind, astute, and sympathetic, he has been unfailingly helpful and open-minded at every step along the way. We count ourselves fortunate to have had the great pleasure of working with him on this book. Among the many others at Duke whose efforts contributed significantly to producing this book, we want to acknowledge Willa Armstrong, Amy Ruth Buchanan, Katie Courtland, Michael McCullough, and Jessica Ryan. For additional editorial and organizational help in preparing the manuscript we are grateful to Carmen Merport, José Medina, Sarah Tuohey, Cathryn Bearov, Aleks Prigozhin, and the crack indexer Scott Smiley.

As we worked on this book, we had the benefit of input from a number of readers whose generous responses were both enlightening and transformative. Leo Bersani and Amy Villarejo revealed themselves after the fact to have been the strong-minded and perceptive anonymous evaluators who read the text for Duke, and we want to express our appreciation for the care that went into their responses. We would also like to thank the many University of Chicago faculty and students who participated in the manuscript reading workshop at the Center for the Study of Gender and Sexuality. Special thanks for extended conversation about the project go to Lisa Ruddick, D. A. Miller, Anjali Arondekar, Candace Vogler, and Ian Horswill. And for his outstanding skills as a reader, among so many other things too numerous (or too intimate) to mention here, we want to thank Joseph Litvak.

REFERENCES

Ahmed, Sara. 2010. *The Promise of Happiness*. Durham: Duke University Press.

Armantrout, Rae. 2010. *Versed*. Middletown, Conn.: Wesleyan University Press.

Badiou, Alain. (1998) 2001. *Ethics: An Essay on the Understanding of Evil*. Trans. Peter Hallward. New York: Verso.

Barthes, Roland. (1977) 1979. *A Lover's Discourse*. Trans. Richard Howard. New York: Hill and Wang.

Berardi, Franco. 2009. *Precarious Rhapsody*. Ed. Erik Empson and Stevphen Shukaitis. Trans. Arianna Bove, Michael Goddard, Giuseppina Mecchia, Antonella Schintu, and Steve Wright. London: Minor Compositions.

Berlant, Lauren. 2011. *Cruel Optimism*. Durham: Duke University Press.

———. 2009. "Neither Monstrous nor Pastoral, but Scary and Sweet: Some Thoughts on Sex and Emotional Performance in *Intimacies* and *What Do Gay Men Want?*" *Women and Performance* 19 (2): 261–73.

———. 2008. *The Female Complaint: The Unfinished Business of Sentimentality in American Culture*. Durham: Duke University Press.

———. 2007. "Starved." *South Atlantic Quarterly* 106 (3): 433–44.

———. 1997. *The Queen of America Goes to Washington City: Essays on Sex and Citizenship*. Durham: Duke University Press.

Bersani, Leo. 2010. *Is the Rectum a Grave? And Other Essays*. Chicago: University of Chicago Press.

Bersani, Leo, and Adam Phillips. 2008. *Intimacies*. Chicago: University of Chicago Press.

Blake, William. 2008. *The Complete Poetry and Prose of William Blake*. Ed. David Erdman. Berkeley: University of California Press.

Bollas, Christopher. 1987. *The Shadow of the Object: Psychoanalysis of the Unthought Known*. New York: Columbia University Press.

Butler, Judith. 2004. *Precarious Life: The Powers of Mourning and Violence*. London: Verso.

Caserio, Robert L., Lee Edelman, Judith Halberstam, José Esteban Muñoz, and Tim Dean. 2006. "The Antisocial Thesis in Queer Theory." PMLA 121 (3): 819–28.

Cavell, Stanley. 1997. *Contesting Tears: The Hollywood Melodrama of the Unknown Woman*. Chicago: University of Chicago Press.

———. 1984. *Pursuits of Happiness: The Hollywood Comedy of Remarriage*. Cambridge: Harvard University Press.

Davis, Lydia. 2010. *The Collected Stories of Lydia Davis*. New York: Picador.

Dean, Jodi. 2010. *Blog Theory: Feedback and Capture in the Circuits of Drive*. London: Polity Press.

de Lauretis, Teresa. 2011. "Queer Texts, Bad Habits, and the Issue of a Future." *GLQ: A Journal of Lesbian and Gay Studies* 17 (2–3): 243–63.

de Man, Paul. 1986. "The Resistance to Theory." In *The Resistance to Theory*. Minneapolis: University of Minnesota Press.

———. 1979. *Allegories of Reading: Figural Language in Rousseau, Nietzsche, Rilke, and Proust*. New Haven: Yale University Press.

Dumm, Thomas. 2008. *Loneliness as a Way of Life*. Cambridge: Harvard University Press.

Edelman, Lee. 2011. "Against Survival: Queerness in a Time That's out of Joint." *Shakespeare Quarterly* 62 (2): 148–69.

———. 2004. *No Future: Queer Theory and the Death Drive*. Durham: Duke University Press.

Freud, Sigmund. (1920) 1955. *Beyond the Pleasure Principle*. In *The Standard Edition of the Complete Psychological Works of Sigmund Freud*, vol. 18. Ed. James Strachey. London: Hogarth Press.

Frost, Robert. 1995. *Robert Frost: Collected Poems, Prose, and Plays*. Ed. Richard Poirier and Mark Richardson. New York: Library of America.

Hardt, Michael, and Antonio Negri. 2012. *Declaration*. New York: Argo-Navis.

Hocquenghem, Guy. (1972) 1993. *Homosexual Desire*. Durham: Duke University Press.

Johnson, Barbara. 1987. *A World of Difference*. Baltimore: Johns Hopkins University Press.

Lacan, Jacques. (1991) 2007. *The Other Side of Psychoanalysis. The Seminar of Jacques Lacan, Book XVII*. Ed. Jacques-Alain Miller. Trans. Russell Griggs. New York: Norton.

———. (1986) 1992. *The Ethics of Psychoanalysis, 1959–1960. The Seminar of Jacques Lacan, Book VII*. Ed. Jacques-Alain Miller. Trans. Dennis Potter. New York: Norton.

———. (1975) 1988. *Freud's Papers on Technique 1953–1954. The Seminar of Jacques Lacan Book I*. Ed. Jacques-Alain Miller. Trans. John Forrester. Cambridge: Cambridge University Press.

———. (1973) 1978. *The Four Fundamental Concepts of Psycho-Analysis. The Seminar of Jacques Lacan Book XI*. Ed. Jacques-Alain Miller. Trans. Alan Sheridan. Norton.

———. (1966) 2006. *Écrits: The First Complete Edition in English*. Trans. Bruce Fink. New York: Norton.

Laplanche, Jean. 1999. *Essays on Otherness*. Ed. and trans. John Fletcher. New York: Routledge.

Laplanche, Jean, and J.-B. Pontalis. 1968. "Fantasy and the Origins of Sexuality." *International Journal of Psychoanalysis* 49: 1–18.

Miller, D. A. 2005. *Jane Austen, or The Secret of Style*. Princeton: Princeton University Press.

Moten, Fred, and Stefano Harney. N.d. "Policy." Center for Research Architecture, http://roundtable.kein.org/node/1164.

Nancy, Jean-Luc. 2003. "Shattered Love." In *A Finite Thinking*. Trans. Simon Sparks. Palo Alto: Stanford University Press.

Ngai, Sianne. 2005. "The Cuteness of the Avant-Garde." *Critical Inquiry* 31, no. 4: 811–47.

Nietzsche, Friedrich. (1954) 1976. *Twilight of the Idols*. In *The Portable Nietzsche*. Ed. and trans. Walter Kaufmann. New York: Penguin Books.

Phillips, Adam. 1994. "Freud and the Uses of Forgetting." In *On Flirtation: Psychoanalytic Essays on the Uncommitted Life*. Cambridge: Harvard University Press.

———. 1993. "Plotting for Kisses." In *On Kissing, Tickling, and Being Bored: Psychoanalytic Essays on the Unexamined Life*. Cambridge: Harvard University Press.

Proulx, Annie. 1999. "Brokeback Mountain." In *Close Range: Wyoming Stories*. New York: Scribner.

Rancière, Jacques. 2009. *Aesthetics and Its Discontents*. Trans. Steven Corcoran. Malden, Mass.: Polity Press.

Rankine, Claudia. 2004. *Don't Let Me Be Lonely: An American Lyric*. Minneapolis: Greywolf Press.

Rickels, Laurence. 1996. "Silent Reading." In *Larry Johnson*. Ed. Scott Watson. Vancouver: Morris and Helen Belkin Art Gallery, University of British Columbia. http://hydra.humanities.uci.edu/twd/cute2.html.

Rubin, Gayle. 2011. "Thinking Sex." In *Deviations: A Gayle Rubin Reader*. Durham: Duke University Press.

Salecl, Renata. 2004. "Love Anxieties." In *On Anxiety*. New York: Routledge.

Samuels, Andrew. 1997. "New Developments in the Post-Jungian Field." In *The Cambridge Companion to Jung*. Ed. Polly Young-Eisendrath and Terence Dawson. New York: Cambridge University Press.

Sedgwick, Eve Kosofsky. 2011. *The Weather in Proust*. Ed. Jonathan Goldberg. Durham: Duke University Press.

REFERENCES

———. 2007. "Melanie Klein and the Difference Affect Makes." *South Atlantic Quarterly* 106 (3): 625–42.

———. 2003. *Touching Feeling: Affect, Pedagogy, Performativity.* Durham: Duke University Press.

———. 2000. *A Dialogue on Love.* Boston: Beacon Press.

———. 1993. "White Glasses." In *Tendencies.* Durham: Duke University Press.

Seltzer, Mark. 1998. *Serial Killers: Death and Life in America's Wound Culture.* London: Routledge.

Sontag, Susan, with Howard Hodgkin. 1991. *The Way We Live Now.* London: Jonathan Cape.

Spivak, Gayatri Chakravorty. 1987. *In Other Worlds: Essays In Cultural Politics.* London: Routledge.

Stevens, Wallace. (1954) 1990. *The Collected Poems of Wallace Stevens.* New York: Vintage Books.

Wittig, Monique. 1992. *The Straight Mind: And Other Essays.* Boston: Beacon Press.

Wordsworth, William. 2004. *Selected Poems.* New York: Penguin Books.

Žižek, Slavoj. 2000. *The Ticklish Subject: The Absent Center of Political Ontology.* New York: Verso.

Filmography

July, Miranda, director. 2005. *Me and You and Everyone We Know.*

Mitchell, John Cameron, director. 2006. *Shortbus.*

Ray, Nicholas, director. 1956. *Bigger Than Life.*

INDEX

....

Note: page numbers in *italics* refer to illustrations; those followed by "n" indicate endnotes.

7; misrepresentation and, 68–69; negativity and, viii–ix, xvii; non-sovereignty and, x, 98, 99, 105–6; as "scene" or "site," 106–7

Coppertone girl, 33

cruising, 99, 103

crush, 80, 81–82

curation, in *Me and You and Everyone We Know*, 25–27

cuteness, 17, 33

Davis, Lydia: "Center of the Story," 103, 107; *Collected Stories*, xvi; "How Shall I Mourn Them," 102–3, 108. *See also* "Break It Down" (Davis)

death: in *Me and You and Everyone We Know*, 22, 24, 27; Panoptimism and, 19; Sedgwick on, 45

death drive, 18, 19, 28, 61, 69–70

decision, drama of, 95–96

dedramatization, 6, 9, 13–14, 65

de Lauretis, Teresa, 70, 71, 87

de Man, Paul, 31, 98

depressive position, 39, 41–42, 52

Descartes, René, 86

desire: anal, 33; the beautiful and, 15–16; comedy and, 31; Davis's "Break It Down" and, 92, 99, 102; dedramatization and, 13; dialogue and, 68; dread and, 39, 53, 54; the drive and, 91, 98; the encounter and, 121, 124; fantasy and, 94, 97, 107; for nonsovereignty, 117; optimism and, 6; representation and, 63–64; Sedgwick and, 45, 49, 51–52, 55; unknowability and, 63–64

detachment, 11–12, 17, 50–51, 53, 56

dialogue. *See* conversation or dialogue

A Dialogue on Love (Sedgwick), 39–41, 50–51, 53, 55–56, 59

digitality, Sedgwick on, 42–43, 48

disavowal: acknowledgment and, 83–84; desire and, 92; dread and, 47, 49–50; fetish and, 79–80, 82, 86, 89, 98; futurity and, 116; of negativity, 14, 64; optimism and, ix

divorce, in *Me and You and Everyone We Know*, 24

domination, 123–24

Don't Let Me Be Lonely (Rankine), 37–38

drama: acknowledgment of, 67; of decision, 95–96; dedramatization, 13–14, 65; melodrama, 50–51; misrecognition and, 65–67; Sedgwick and, 50–58; staging and, 57; "stopping," 56–57

dread, 39–40, 49–50, 53, 54, 59–60

the drive: change of scene and, 107; circuit of, 63; community, division, and, 109; dedramatization and, 14; desire and, 64, 94, 98; irreducible otherness and, 69; negativity and, 29, 95, 120; nonsovereignty and, 112, 113; queer negativity, political thought, and, 70–72; rethinking and, 8

Dumm, Tom, 37–38

Ehrenreich, Barbara, 20

encounter: affect and, 76; attunement and, 110; change and, 89, 92, 100, 108, 112; dialogue and, ix–x, 69; the drive and, 120; impossibility of, 95, 113–14; incoherence and traumatic encounters, 8–11; meanings of, viii, 109; nonrelation and, 28, 90, 105; parsing problem of defining, 74–75; "surprise of otherness" and, xi; the unbearable and, 35, 69, 90, 97, 113, 120; as undoing of sovereignty, 2,

Sedgwick, Eve Kosofsky (*continued*)
45–46; "Melanie Klein and the
Difference Affect Makes," 41–42,
46, 48, 49–50, 52; on necessity
and nonnecessity, 54–55; negativity, repair, and, xv; "Paranoid
Reading and Reparative Reading," 41–44, 57; "The Pedagogy
of Buddhism," 45–46; possible
vs. impossible and, 58–59; "The
Weather in Proust," 47–48, 51–53;
"White Glasses," 49
Seltzer, Mark, 40
sex: the aesthetic as inseparable
from, 15; calculable or incalcula-
ble, 75, 80; critical neglect of, 63;
as drive, 91; as encounter divorced
from meaning making, 11–12, 93;
meanings of, 7, 26; mobility and
attachment, 63, 91; shock of discontinuity and encounter with
nonknowledge, 4, 71; as site for
encountering negativity, 1–2, 15,
31–32, 63, 113, 116–17; as sublime
vs. beautiful, 15–17; as syncopation, 55–56; as tragicomic conversation, 113–14. *See also* "Break It
Down" (Davis); encounter
"sexual outlaws," 4–5
sexual revolution, math of, 101
sex without optimism: adorabil-
ity, cuteness, and, 15–18, 32–33;
comparison of examples of, 7–10,
14–15; comparison of idioms
around, 4–7, 10–14; happiness
and, 18–20; in Johnson's *Untitled
(Ass)*, 16, 28–33; in July's *Me and
You and Everyone We Know*, 20–28;
Lacan's "there is no sexual relation" and, 1–2; negativity and, 2–3;
optimism and negativity, oscillation between, 33–34; responses to

phrase, 1; story, education, and,
3–4, 5; togetherness and, 1
shame, 37, 39
shock, 4, 6, 8–9, 15
sinthomosexual, 18
skeleton in Davis's "Break It Down,"
74, 78, 86–87
Sontag, Susan, 27
sovereignty: encounter as undoing
of, 2, 29, 54, 64–69, 97; in expectation of nonsovereignty, 120; fantasy of, 97; Ovid's Pygmalion and,
31. *See also* nonsovereignty
Spivak, Gayatri Chakravorty, 92
"staying bound to a world," 20,
28–29
Stevens, Wallace, 70
The Straight Mind (Wittig), 14
structure: change, negativity, and,
121; fantasy and, 67, 88–89,
93–94; as process vs. imprint of
production of life, 12; sex without
optimism and, 7–8, 10–11; transformation, constraints on, 69–70
style, 80–82
stylothete, 81
surprise, xi, 4, 15, 117, 120–21
survival: abandonment, 40–41, 56;
dread, 39–40, 49–50, 53, 54,
59–60; failure and, 37; karma,
reincarnation, and the Buddhist
nonself and, 45–46, 51–53; loneliness, 37–41; loss and, 47, 48;
paranoia and, 41–44. *See also* reparativity
symptoms, 55
syncopation, 56
systems, open vs. closed, 48, 51

teleology, 33, 70, 108
theory, 71, 87, 98
togetherness, 1

Tomkins, Silvan, xv

transformation: acknowledgment and, 86; affective, possibilities of, 67, 69, 83–84; disturbance and, xvii; encounter with negativity and, 18; *Me and You and Everyone We Know* and, 26; negativity and, 29; Sedgwick on, 51, 52; structural constraints on, 69–70; utopianism and, 64

trumping, 53–54, 58

the unbearable: as ambivalence, 61; conversation and, 105; encounter and, 35, 69, 90, 97, 113, 120; enjoyment and, vii, 9, 32, 90; negativity and, 67, 94, 121; the otherness that permits no relation, 98, 105, 107–8; pleasure in structure of, 90–91, 117; reiteration of, 121; relationality and, 27, 54–55, 122, 124; world building and, 89, 112, 121–22

undoing: change as, 107; of control, 32–33; in Davis's "Center of the Story," 103; interpretations of, 64–65; of love, 59; optimism and,

18–19; resistance and, 115; sex without optimism and, 7–8. See *also* sex without optimism

unruliness of the world, 83

the unthought known, 90, 96

Untitled (Ass) (Johnson), 16, 29–33, 115

utopianism, 5, 11, 64

vacations, 100–101

Versed (Armantrout), 37–38

violence, 17, 18, 32, 50, 112, 115

wanting, 36, 42–43

"The Weather in Proust" (Sedgwick), 47–48, 51–53

"White Glasses" (Sedgwick), 49

Wilden, Anthony, 43

witness, 27, 50–51

Wittig, Monique, 14

Wordsworth, William, 15

world-building, 9, 15, 89, 110–12, 121–22

worlding, 89, 100, 107, 111, 112

zingers, 40, 57

Žižek, Slavoj, 94